Live Healthy

Now & Forever!

Learn how to get healthy and stay healthy the holistic, natural way – right now! Jeffrey Laign shows readers the road to good health and long life by applying the intelligent use of herbs, supplements, nutrition, exercise, mind and spirit. Each chapter features practical advice, lots of useful tips, straight talk about health and modern medicine, and an action plan to start you on your way. And there's also a unique Appendix showing you how to best prevent and treat various problems, including sore throats, muscle pain, insomnia, arthritis, toothaches, sunburns and much more.

About the Author

JEFFREY LAIGN has written and contributed to many books on health, nutrition and exercise, including *How to Heal Yourself, Slow Down Aging,* and *Nature's Miracle Medicines.* A leading medical journalist, Laign has gathered roots in China with traditional healers, interviewed Indian medicine men in the Amazon, explored the healing benefits of saunas in Lapland, and pored through barks and leaves with South African tribal healers. For 10 years he was managing editor of publications at Health Communications, a leading publisher of wellness books; while there he played a key role in developing the best-seller *Chicken Soup for the Soul.* He was a staff writer for *Your Health* magazine and has produced five bimonthly magazines covering body, mind and spirit. He lives in Ft. Lauderdale, Florida.

Live Healthy
Now & Forever!

Jeffrey Laign

Cold Spring Press

Cold Spring Press

P.O. Box 284, Cold Spring Harbor, NY 11724
E-mail: Jopenroad@aol.com

Copyright©2003 by Jeffrey Laign
All Rights Reserved

ISBN 1-892975-97-1
Library of Congress Control Number: 2003104439

Table of Contents

Appendix   143

Index   161

Sidebars

–Action Plans in Bold for Easy Reference–

Live Healthy Now & Forever!

Introduction

It Ain't Rocket Science

It's easy to achieve good health. Making just a few simple changes in your lifestyle will do wonders for your body, mind and spirit.

I am not a doctor. I don't even play one on TV. Then how dare I presume to offer you advice on achieving and maintaining good health? Everyone knows, after all, that self-help books must be written by experts, right?

Well, I am not an expert. I am just like you, an average person who wants to feel better and live life to the fullest but is baffled more often than not by our country's budget-shattering, mazelike healthcare system, seemingly contradictory scientific studies and mountains of pills, potions and prescriptions, all of which promise to grant us a long, happy life.

As a journalist who has covered a wide range of health issues, I have interviewed scores of doctors, scientists, nutritionists, pharmacists and psychologists. Over the years they have offered me hundreds of opinions, beliefs and "facts" about healing body, mind and spirit. I offer you those insights here—and, make no mistake, this expert advice is sensible and sound.

But I also want you to realize that to enjoy good health you needn't rely solely on the advice of experts. I want you to know that you can take charge of your life and give yourself the gift of good health. It's easier and far simpler than you may have imagined.

Why do we look to experts to solve our problems? In our increasingly complex society, life can be difficult, and we tend to make it more so. Put

13

two people in a room and sooner or later one of them will begin devising rules and bylaws. Before you know it you've got an organization. Put three people in a room and eventually you will have the National Institutes of Health.

Good health requires no institutions. It's nature, not rocket science. You don't need to employ a chef with five degrees in nutritional science to prepare every morsel you pop in your mouth (unless you're Oprah—and I'm pretty sure you're not). You don't need to mortgage your house to hire a personal trainer, nor is it necessary for you to devote half of your waking hours to punishing yourself compulsively in a gym. You don't need to give up French fries and subsist on rice cakes or carrot sticks. You don't have to give up anything, in fact.

Take a cue from your pets. I'll bet your dog, for the most part, is pretty darn healthy. That's because he eats when he's hungry, and consumes only what his body needs for fuel. He gets plenty of exercise, but only as much as his body requires to keep his heart healthy and his muscles primed. Your cat as well may have more common sense than many humans. She sleeps when her body needs to rest and restore itself. She doesn't work herself to death behind a desk or fret about circumstances she is powerless to change. Heck, a big part of her life is spent just having fun, even if it's only batting a ball of twine.

Modern-Day Methusalahs

Why bother to improve your health? If you read a newspaper or watch TV, you may suspect from time to time that the world is poised on the brink of Armageddon. Trust me (even though I'm not an expert) that the world is not going to end tomorrow and neither are you. In fact, you're likely to go on breathing for a long, long time.

"Americans on average are living longer than ever before," says Health and Human Services Secretary Tommy G. Thompson. "Much of this is due to the progress we've made in fighting diseases that account for a majority of deaths in the country."

The Centers for Disease Control reports that average life expectancy for Americans in 2000 was 76.9 years, up from 76.7 years in 1999, and most experts agree that numbers will continue to climb.

"Two-thirds of all men and women who have lived beyond the age of 65 in the entire history of the world are alive today," says aging expert Ken Dychtwald.

Sociologists estimate that by 2025 there will be 822 million people in the world who are 65 and older—a number greater than the current combined populations of Europe and North America. But don't stop at 65.

INTRODUCTION

Centenarians used to be extremely rare. Now there are more than 45,000 Americans over the age of 100. Trend watcher Cheryl Russell predicts that 1 million Baby Boomers will reach the century mark

Why are we living longer? Certainly genes play a role. Gerontologists credit "good genes" with extending the life span of Jeanne Louise Calment, a French woman who lived to be 122, even though she smoked, drank and ate whatever she pleased.

"We know that specific genes are involved in aging," says Roy L. Walford, M.D., professor of pathology at UCLA.

As we continue to unlock the longevity secrets of genes, it's only a matter of time before science is able extend our lives by "manipulating" basic DNA. That's already happening, in fact.

Fruit flies have lived well beyond expectation after researchers tinkered with their genetic makeup. Even more promising are studies of a worm that can "stop time." When *Caenorhabditis elegans* is under environmental stress, it enters a state of hibernation known as the dauer stage. The worm stops eating, stores fat instead of metabolizing it, and thus lengthens its life from two weeks to two months or more.

In 1997 Boston scientist Gary Ruvkun and colleagues reported success at cloning the worm's longevity gene. Moreover, the researchers discovered that the gene could be manipulated to halt or enhance the worm's ability to enter the dauer phase and extend its life.

"The goal would be to induce a metabolically efficient state in humans that's similar to the worm's dauer stage," says Michael Jazwinski, Ph.D., a geneticist at Louisiana State University Medical Center in New Orleans

But what about those of us with "bad" or "average" genes? Must we wait for science to "fix" us or resign ourselves to early graves? Not at all. Mounting evidence indicates that genes aren't the only factor that determines health and longevity.

For years, researchers have thought that many adult health problems were "predetermined." According to the Fetal Origins of Adult Disease Hypothesis, formulated in 1986, we may be "destined" to get sick because of conditions that occurred before we were born.

The theory holds that if a fetus does not receive the nourishment it needs, it diverts available nutrients to areas that require immediate attention, such as the brain. In doing so, the fetus deprives other organs, such as the heart or lungs. This rerouting of resources may change the baby's biological structure, functioning and metabolism, making it more vulnerable than normal to develop certain diseases as an adult. Some scientists, for example, long have suspected a correlation between low birth weight and high blood pressure later in life.

But a new study led by Oxford University researcher Rory Collins questions whether that link is as strong as we have believed. "Surprisingly this hypothesis doesn't seem to have gone through rigorous scrutiny," Collins says in the British medical journal *The Lancet*. "It seems to have been adopted very widely, very rapidly, without too much in the way of critical appraisal."

Do it Yourself

Even if you were deprived of nutrients as a fetus, even if you have bad genes, there's still hope for living a long, healthy life. Take a tip from Thompson. "We can do more by eating right, exercising regularly and taking other simple steps to promote good health and prevent serious illness and disease."

What's more, you don't require an organization, institution or expert to guide you. Come on, do you really need the government to warn you that smoking is bad for your health? Take charge of your health and do it today. In this book you'll find me expanding on the following advice:

•Eat better. That doesn't mean you have to give up everything you enjoy. Wolf down a Big Mac from time to time, Just don't have one for lunch every day. Don't think you can lose weight by gorging on fat-free foods. They do more harm than good. Have a slice of pizza now and then, but for the most part go for good, wholesome foods, including lean meats and fresh fruits and vegetables.
•Shop at Mother Nature's pharmacy. Try herbs and natural supplements. Ever notice that when your dog is a little under the weather he nibbles grass? Visit a health-food store or talk with your pharmacist about natural nutrients that can help you to feel better and look years younger.
•Exercise regularly, but take it easy. Don't try to whip yourself into shape. You don't need a model's body—and why would you want to look like a toothpick anyway? Excessive exercise can be more harmful than none at all. Just 20 minutes a day may be all you require for good health.
•Nourish your mind and spirit, as well as your body. Meditate, relax, read something uplifting or educational every day.
•Explore natural therapies to maintain you're health. Try acupuncture, yoga or Ayurveda.
•Don't forget to have fun. As your cat would tell you if she could, there's no use in having good health if you don't enjoy life.

If you incorporate even some of these changes in your life you will feel better. That's a promise. Will you live as long as a biblical patriarch? "I don't think we can live forever," says John Wilmoth, assistant professor of demography at UCLA in Berkeley, California. "But we haven't been able to find a fixed limit for the human life span."

It's important to know that you don't have to be perfect in your pursuit of the good life (unless you are Martha Stewart—and I am *certain* that you are not). I am not perfect. Not by a long shot. Like most people, I am a mass of contradictions. I practice yoga, ride my bicycle and try to eat as many fresh fruits and vegetables as possible. On the other hand, I sometimes indulge in "forbidden" foods (Whopper with cheese, please). I have from time to time imbibed more than the recommended single glass of wine a day and on occasion I've been observed to light up a Dominican cigar after a particularly satisfying meal.

Healthy? Of course not. Human? You bet. The point I'm trying to make is that good health is a process and you have the rest of your life to work on it. In the meantime, despite periodic lapses—and you will have them—you will feel and look far better than you have in years.

Remember, health is a journey, not a destination. Live healthy, now and forever. Begin your journey today.

—Jeffrey Laign
Fort Lauderdale, Florida
August, 2003

1. Nutrition

Fuel up For Fitness

The food that you put in your body determines, to a large extent, the level of health you can expect to attain.

Munch a handful of honey-roasted almonds. Sip a glass of red wine. Indulge yourself with a chocolate kiss. You're already eating healthier.

That's right. Many of the treats you may have denied yourself actually are good for you. Scientists at the University of Illinois have found that honey contains the same level of health-giving antioxidants as many fruits and vegetables, such as spinach, strawberries, oranges, bananas and apples.

"People could incorporate honey in places where they might be using some sort of sweetening agent, like sugar, and this might contribute a significant amount of (antioxidants)," says lead researcher Nicki Engeseth, Ph.D.

Wine as well is good for you. Take a look at France. Renowned for its mouthwatering, artery-clogging cheeses, France boasts one of the world's lowest rates of heart disease. Why? Nutritionists think it's because French diners often enjoy antioxidant-rich red wine with meals.

What's more, we now know that chocolate—thank the Universe—is chock-full of feel-good chemicals than can help to lift our spirits and regulate our moods. Food scientists are even looking at whether some compounds in chocolate actually may prolong our lives.

So why have we spent so many years shunning foods such as these? Perhaps we imagined that if we gave them up, along with butter, meat, bread—everything that tastes good—we might live forever. Even if we

18

could, who would want to if we had to subsist on fat-free cookies, fat-free chips, fat-free crackers, tasteless rice cakes, chemical-laden margarines? We might as well eat the stuffing of a bean-bag chair.

Even worse than munching on dormitory furniture is starving yourself to attain a model-thin physique. If you're doing that you're way off base. More and more studies are concluding that diets that deny simply don't work.

Then what does? How can we eat real food and maintain a healthy weight? Our great grandparents never asked that question. They'd probably be amazed, in fact, to learn that something as ostensibly simple as eating has become such a complex issue. But these days, when food scientists seem to contradict themselves every other day, it *is* hard to know how eat.

Only a few years ago, for example, nutritionists recommended that we load up on carbohydrates such as pasta and rice. Now Dr. Atkins urges us to cut the carbs and fill our plates with proteins and—gulp—fats. What's a diner to do?

> *Stop obsessing about food. Have your cake and eat it too. Just don't go hog wild. And be sure to take advantage of the healing properties inherent in most foods.*

The Best Medicine

Believe it or not, the foods you buy each week at the grocery store are potent medicines. Mounting research indicates that the foods we put in our bodies may cause and cure many of the ailments that plague us. That's because they're packed with "phytochemicals" that profoundly affect every one of our biological systems.

"Diet is more powerful than we ever thought it to be," says Neal Barnard, M.D., author of several best-selling books on nutrition, including *Food for Life*. "We can use diet to reverse heart disease and cut our cancer risk in half. And the foods we eat affect our moods as well as our physiological functions. Food are extraordinary allies in our wars on disease. There is nothing speculative or far-out about that premise."

Scientists have not identified all of the thousands of phytochemicals that offer protection against diseases, such as cancer. "But we don't need years of research," says Gabriel Feldman, M.D., who has worked as the American Cancer Society's director of prostate and colorectal cancer. "If people would implement what we know today, cancer rates would drop. It's that simple."

Foods also are important when it comes to fighting pain. Olive oil, a staple of the much-touted Mediterranean diet, not only offers protection against heart disease but also helps to ease pain, including some symptoms associated with menopause.

"When your body is starved of fat, it shuts down reproductive functions," says Laurence M. Demers, Ph.D., professor of pathology and medicine at Penn State's Milton S. Hershey Medical Center. " Therefore, you need a certain percentage of body fat to bring about normal hormone production for normal menstrual regularity."

Several other foods are important medicines for women. Calcium is essential during and after menopause. An extra glass of skim milk or a cup of collard greens—chock full of calcium—may help to prevent mood swings and menstrual pain, as well as osteoporosis, says U.S. Dept. of Agriculture expert James G. Penland, Ph. D.

Kick Cancer in the Crotch

OK, here's the bad news: Each year prostate cancer strikes more than 200,000 American men—and what you eat may determine how likely you are to get it.

"Cancer of the prostate is strongly linked to what men eat," says nutritionist Neal Barnard, M.D. "The prostate is very sensitive to hormones. Men who consume diets based on animal products tend to have more testosterone and estrogens, compared to men who eat healthier diets. The higher levels of these hormones make them the chief suspects in the epidemic of prostate cancer."

Now here's the good news. New studies prove what guys have always known: Pizza—one of mankind's most important food groups—is good for us. Mounting research suggests. that phytochemicals found in tomato sauce and other foods may play a pivotal role in putting the brakes on prostate cancer.

Tomatoes contain lycopene, a potent antioxidant. "The lycopene is better absorbed if it's in cooked or processed tomatoes, compared to eating fresh tomatoes," says researcher Omer Kucuk, M.D., who observed the effects of lycopene among 33 prostate-cancer patients at Karmanos Cancer Institute in Detroit.

And the news gets better, says physician and best-selling author Andrew Weil. "Fat must be present for lycopene to be absorbed." So don't forget to load that marinara sauce with good old olive oil.

And don't forget soybeans. They're high in phytoestrogens and can do a great deal to ease change-of-life symptoms. Soybeans also may provide protection against breast cancer and other forms of this devastating disease. But when was the last time you had soybeans for dinner?

Americans die of breast, colon and prostate cancers at five to 30 times the rate of people in other parts of the world. That may be because Americans tend to avoid super-healthy foods like soybeans and chow down on additive-packed fast foods. Nearly a third of all cancers, in fact, may result from poor diets, say scientists at the World Cancer Research Fund and the American Institute for Cancer Research.

"It has now been well accepted that proper nutrition could prevent from 50 percent to 90 percent of all cancers," says Patrick Quillin, Ph.D., author of *Beating Cancer with Nutrition.*

Eating nutritious foods could reduce cancer rates dramatically, Quillin says. A study of 14,000 Seventh-Day Adventists, in fact, found that men who regularly ate beans, lentils, tomatoes, raisins, dates and dried fruit enjoyed a reduced incidence of prostate cancer.

> *Adding wholesome foods to your diet is the easiest way to get healthy and stay that way.*

Fill 'er Up

It's a tired but true analogy: Your body is like your car—it needs good fuel to run. "But many people," says Barnard, "put the wrong fuel in their bodies—foods that clog their arteries, push hormones out of balance, irritate their tissues and cause gradually worsening pain. They will never know how good their bodies can feel until they find the right foods and their healing begins. It can be like having a brand-new body."

Consider this: A study published recently in the *Journal of the American Medical Association,* found that women who ate diets rich in fruits, vegetables, whole grains and lean meats were 30 percent less likely to die of any cause than women whose diets were not as rich in nutrients.

Sound simple? It is. Cooking and eating healthy foods is fun—and surprisingly easy. "Ten years ago," Barnard says, "health-food stores were dingy little places with dusty products and a guy behind the counter in a tie-dyed shirt named Sunshine. Now health-food stores are the size of grocery stores and they offer all kinds of products. What's more, these products actually taste good. They've risen in quality dramatically and prices are starting to come down." Consider some of the healthy options awaiting you.

Eat Your Veggies

Your mother may have been wrong about a lot of things, but not about vegetables. They really are good for you. Take a look at the medical benefits you may derive from chowing down on:

Artichokes. They contain a chemical called cynarin, which may help to lower cholesterol.

Carrots. Rich in antioxidants alphacarotene and betacarotene, carrots are providing food for thought for scientists looking to prevent cancer.

Celery. Crunch a stalk to derive the benefits of psoralens. These chemicals may protect against lymphoma.

Chili peppers. Pop a hot one. A new study at the University of Texas MD Anderson Cancer Center in Houston reports that capsaicin—the chemical that makes chilis hot—and a related compound called reinferatoxin starve cancer cells of oxygen, forcing them to self-destruct.

Cruciferous vegetables. Have second servings of broccoli, cauliflower and cabbage. They contain sulforaphane, which boosts production of enzymes that wash away chemical debris and may stop some carcinogens in their tracks, says Johns Hopkins pharmacologist Paul Talalay, M.D.

Kale. May not be the most popular part of your dinner, but it should be. Kale contains the cancer-fighting antioxidants lutein and zeaxanthin.

Legumes. Beans, in other words. They're high in complex carbohydrates, fiber and quality proteins, and they're free of cholesterol. Beans are great for diabetics because they have a remarkable balancing effect on insulin that lasts for hours. And some beans, notably soybeans and derivative products such as tofu and tempeh, contain "many potentially beneficial compounds that may help to prevent certain types of cancer," says pharmacist and best-selling author Earl Mindell, Ph.D. Soy, for example, contains genistein, which appears to prevent cancerous tumors from growing. Soy products also contain isoflavones, which may reduce risk of breast and ovarian cancers; phytosterols, which slow reproduction of cancer cells in the large intestine, helping to prevent colon cancer; protease inhibitors, which suppress production of certain enzymes in cancer cells and may slow tumor growth; and saponins, which block abnormal processes by which DNA reproduces, thus preventing cancer cells from multiplying.

Onions. They're worth crying over. Onions, garlic and chives are full of allyl sulfides, which help the body to process cancer-causing chemicals. Allyl sulfides also increase production of glutathione S-transferase, a chemical that makes it easier for the body to excrete carcinogens. In addition, allium compounds have natural antibiotic properties, and help to lower cholesterol and blood pressure. "Even modest amounts in the diet have a marked impact on metabolism," says Pennsylvania State University nutritionist John Milner.

Potatoes. Mashed, boiled or baked, they'll give you catechols, which boost immune function, helping you to fight off illnesses.

Pumpkins. Throw out the jack o' lantern but keep the stuff inside. Pumpkins, like carrots and sweet potatoes, are packed with the cancer-fighting antioxidant betacarotene.

Red bell peppers. Along with tomatoes, these are a good source of lycopene, which wards off prostate cancer.

Spinach. Popeye wasn't fooling. Spinach is good stuff, full of cancer-preventing carotenoids.

Tomatoes. Hard to believe that 16th-century Europeans thought these ruby gems were poisonous. Tomatoes contain more than 10,000 phytochemicals. Besides lycopene, tomatoes offer p-coumaric acid and chlorgenic acid, which neutralizes some cancer-causing chemicals. Moreover, gamma amino butyric acid in tomatoes helps to prevent high blood pressure.

The Meat of the Matter

Load your plate with veggies and you may live longer. As a group, vegetarians have lower blood pressure and cholesterol levels, as well as less incidence of heart disease, osteoporosis, obesity, arthritis, diabetes, kidney disease and certain cancers. "You simply don't need meat to be healthy," says nutritionist and author Suzanne Havala.

Author and nutritional expert Neal Barnard, M.D., says a vegetarian diet may extend your life by roughly a decade. "Your diet," he says, "should be composed primarily of vegetables, fruits, whole grains and legumes. And it's easier than ever to follow a vegetarian diet. You can now find many vegetarian entrees on the menu in most restaurants."

But suppose you don't want to chuck the cheeseburgers and pass the peas? You can still eat meat and enjoy good health. Meat, in fact, is a cornerstone of the popular Atkins diet, which more doctors are recommending. Eat it. Enjoy it. But don't pig out.

As Havala tells clients: "If you can keep your meat intake to a small portion, like a side dish, you're probably all right."

Fabulous Fruits

Fruits didn't do much for Eve, but they will for you. They're tasty and healthy and many may help you to prevent a number of illnesses. Next time you've got the munchies, go for:

Apples. One a day really may keep the doctor away. Apples contain at least six carotenoids that may help to prevent various forms of cancer. You'll benefit from ellagic acid and caffeic acid, which bolster production of enzymes that help your body to wash away carcinogens. Apples also contain ferulic acid, which binds to nitrates in the stomach, blocking them from changing into cancer-causing nitrosamines. And they contain octacosanol, which may increase protection from Parkinson's disease.

Bananas. Packed with immune-boosting catechols, they're appealing indeed. What's more, bananas may help to prevent strokes. A study published recently in the journal *Neurology* found that people with low dietary potassium levels were 1.5 times more likely to suffer a stroke than those who had the highest levels in their diets. Bananas are a good source of dietary potassium, says Deborah M. Green, M.D., who worked on the study at the Neuroscience Institute of The Queen's Medical Center in Honolulu.

Blueberries. They contain anthocyanosides, which may prevent heart disease

Cantaloupes. Put them on a pedestal. Like pumpkins, cantaloupes contain betacarotene, which may help to prevent cancer.

Figs. These feature benzyladehyde, which may prevent cancer, and psoralens, which may help to guard against lymphoma.

Grapes. One study found that reservatrol, an antioxidant found in grapes, reduced the incidence of skin tumors by 88 percent.

Mangoes. Add these to your list of betacarotene-rich fruits.

Oranges. A daily glass of orange juice will give you a healthy shot of vitamin C, a powerful antioxidant that may prevent some forms of cancer. A glass provides twice the folic acid of a navel orange. A pint of juice with lunch will give you half of your daily folic-acid requirement.

Pineapples. They're delicious and they contain an enzyme called bromelain, which may prevent cancer and inflammation. Bromelain also helps with digestive problems.

Strawberries. Like blackberries and raspberries, strawberries contain a number of anticarcinogens, as well as cholorgenic acid, which reduces cholesterol.

Watermelons. Another source of cancer-fighting lycopene.

Fruits and vegetables are among the best food choices, but don't forget that many other options are available to you. For optimal health eat a wide variety of healthful foods.

More Foods to Choose

The best way to lose weight and improve your health is to eat more, not less. Just be sure to pick foods that are good for you—and there are many out there.

Go for Grains

Moderate amounts of grains are essential for good health. Remember that grains are carbohydrates, so don't overdo the servings. But do try these:

Barley, brown rice, corn, and millet. They're packed with fiber, which helps to slow down absorption of glucose in the bloodstream. They may help diabetics to keep blood sugar levels more even.

Oatmeal. The fiber in oatmeal acts like a broom to sweep debris from your digestive tract and prevent colon cancer. "Every spoonful of oatmeal you have for breakfast displaces the eggs and bacon you might otherwise have ingested," says Barnard. Oatmeal offers energy-producing complex carbohydrates and soluble fiber to lower artery-clogging cholesterol, which contributes to illnesses such as heart disease. Oatmeal also contains potent sources of folic acid, which helps to reduce levels of homocysteine, a blood substance that's another indicator of heart disease.

Feel Better With Fish

Americans don't eat enough fish. Cancer levels are remarkably lower in countries like Japan, where fish is a regular part of the diet. Fish, moreover, is good for your heart. *The Journal of the American Medical Association* recently reported that consuming at least one fish meal a week could cut your risk of sudden cardiac death in half.

Best choices are fatty fishes, such as salmon and tuna. These contain omega-3 fatty acids, which have been shown to shrink tumors in rats, says Lillian Thompson, a researcher at the University of Toronto who's studying the nutrient's effects on breast cancer patients. Omega-3 fats may reduce levels of blood triglycerides and provide significant protection from heart disease.

Dealing With Dairy

There are pros and cons of consuming dairy products, such as butter, milk and cheese. Yogurt, for example, contains health-promoting bacteria such as *Lactobacillus bulgaricus*, *Streptococcus thermophilus* and *Lactobacillus acidophilus*, which digest lactose, or milk sugar. They break it down into glucose and galactose, two sugars most adults can absorb. Several European studies indicate that people who eat large amounts of yogurt have a significantly lower risk of developing breast and other cancers.

Milk, moreover, contains significant amounts of calcium, which helps to prevent osteoporosis. The bad news is that milk can cause problems for some people. Most people in the world, for example, are lactose-intolerant. That is, they lack the enzyme needed to process the sugars in milk. Only people of northern-European heritage are genetically programmed to consume cow's milk in large quantities.

But why should they? "Cow's don't drink cow's milk, so why do humans?" asks nutritional writer Harvey Diamond, author (with Marilyn Diamond) of *Fit For Life*. "Cow's milk was designed for one purpose and one only—to feed the young of the species."

Commercially raised cows are fed antibiotics and other chemicals to stimulate growth. Those chemicals inevitably make their way into the milk we drink. In addition, some studies suggest that cow's milk contributes to development of diabetes. That's because milk proteins spur the

Not Milk?

Milk is an excellent source of bone-building calcium. But it's not the only source. You'll also find the mineral in these foods:

Food	mg of calcium
3 ounces calcium-fortified orange juice	100
1/2 oz hard cheese	100
1/4 oz Parmesan	100
1/2 cup yogurt	80-100
1/2 cup macaroni and cheese	80
1/2 packet plain instant oatmeal	80
1 slice processed cheese	60
1/3 cup cream soup	60
1/3 cup spinach	60
1/4 cup broccoli	50
2 dried figs	50
1/4 cup cooked beans	30
1 egg yolk	28
1 oz tofu	27
1 slice bread	25
1/4 cup orange or carrots	15
1/4 cup peas	10

body to produce antibodies that may damage the pancreas. And, of course, dairy products are full of cholesterol and saturated fats.

The bottom line: Don't gulp down gallons of milk or chow down on pounds of cheese. But in moderation, dairy products can play an important role in your healthy diet.

The Skinny on Fat

Fat is the biggest villain since Jesse James. We blame fat for everything—bad hearts, big bellies—and eliminating the stuff from our dinner plates has become almost a national obsession.

But admit it, fat makes everything taste better. The problem is, we're adding the wrong kinds of fats to our diets. Animal fats, saturated fats. They're bad for us.

Scientists from Harvard Medical School and the Harvard School of Public Health spent four years studying the nutritional habits of more than 50,000 male health professionals. The researchers found that men who consumed the most animal fat were nearly twice as likely to develop prostate cancer than were men who ate the least amount.

Even if fat doesn't cause prostate cancer, it may accelerate the illness. At Memorial Sloan-Kettering Cancer Center researchers injected mice with cancerous human prostate cells. They found that mice fed a high-fat diet developed tumors that were two and a half times larger than those found in animals fed a diet low in fat.

Don't think for a minute, though, that you should turn your back on fat. In fact, eat more fat. Just make sure it's the right kind. Go for olive oil, which offers protection against heart disease, and fish like salmon and tuna, which contain healthful omega-3 fatty acids.

"A balance of (fatty acids) is vital to cardiac function, joint health, insulin balance, mood stability, skin health and even gene expression," says Artemis Simopoulous, M.D., editor-in-chief of *World Review of Nutrition and Dietetics* and author of *The Omega Diet.*

"Up until a few years ago," Simopoulous says, "most people had diets that were very balanced in essential fatty acids. Modern diets are really poor."

Salud!

A little booze is not a bad thing. Nutritionists know that red wine is brimming with disease-fighting phytochemicals, which may explain the "French paradox" that enables Gallic diners to consume large quantities of cholesterol-rich butter, cheese and meat while maintaining relatively low levels of heart disease.

French scientists have concluded that moderate amounts of wine not only prevent heart disease but also appear to help those who already have suffered a cardiac attack. In a recent study, middle-age Frenchmen who had suffered one heart attack and drank two or more glasses of wine regularly were 50 percent less likely than nondrinkers to have a second attack. The study was conducted by Dr. Michel de Lorgeril of the Joseph Fourier University of Grenoble, France, and published in *Circulation*, the American Heart Association's journal.

In another study, published in the journal *Epidemiology*, German doctors concluded that drinking beer or wine may stave off ulcers. Researchers at the University of Ulm observed 1,785 men and women ages 18 to 88 and found that the stomachs of beer drinkers contained smaller amounts of ulcer-causing bacteria known as *Helicobacter pylori*; wine drinkers had even less.

German researchers at the University of Dusseldorf followed 66 ulcer patients for a year and discovered, to their surprise, that daily moderate drinking—roughly the amount of alcohol in a shot of spirits—hastened ulcer healing.

The researchers theorized that repeated shots of a mild irritant—a low concentration of alcohol, in other words—strengthen the stomach lining so it can better stand up to attacks by stronger irritants, including stomach acid.

But even if you're attempting to combat gastrointestinal disease, you can't drink till you drop. "Most of the literature suggests that large amounts of beer and wine can damage the stomach lining," says Bennett Roth, M.D., a digestive disease specialist with the University of California, Los Angeles Medical Center.

Tea Time

Coffee give you the jitters? Switch to tea. Green tea contains several antioxidant chemicals known as polyphenols. One compound, called EGCG, has 20 times the free radical-quenching effect of vitamin E, and 500 times the potency of vitamin C. The compound also has been shown to inhibit angiogenesis, the process that stimulates growth of blood vessels. Thus green tea may help to fight tumors, which must form new vessels to grow.

"Green tea is a rich source of polyphenols," says pharmacist and author Mindell. These compounds stimulate detoxifying enzymes that may block cancerous growth, and contain antioxidants more powerful than vitamins C and E.

Unfermented green tea also contains potassium, magnesium and folic acid; catechins, which ward off viral infections and protect against various cancers; and fluoride, which prevents cavities. Some studies also suggest that green tea extract may inhibit the oxidation of LDL, so-called bad cholesterol, and thereby prevent heart disease.

Sweet Dreams

It's no secret that chocolate makes us happy. That's because chocolate's feel-good chemicals include a marijuana-like substance, says Ann E. Kelley, professor of psychiatry at the University of Wisconsin at Madison Medical School. In addition, chocolate contains protein and calcium. The problem is that a one-and-a-half-ounce chocolate bar provides half your daily total of saturated fat. So don't do a Snickers for lunch. But Godiva once in a while? God, yes.

The Diet Dilemma

With all these healthy foods just waiting to be consumed why, then, are we so fat? Americans are known the world over for having big hearts. We're also know for having big bellies and big behinds. A third to half of all Americans, in fact, are considered to be obese, weighing 20 percent more than is ideal for good health.

"As a group, Americans are more overweight than they ever have been," says Barnard. "Fast foods are more ubiquitous than ever. Many people say, I just don't have time to cook healthy meals.'

You have to make time to cook healthy meals. Otherwise, you're going to gain weight and develop health problems. It's as simple as that.

Obesity causes and aggravates a number of life-threatening illnesses, including heart disease, cancer and diabetes. There are many reasons

Calorie Count

Cutting back on calories has been shown to extend life span in nearly all species tested, including invertebrates, fish and mammals, according to the Lifespan Project, directed by Richard Weindruch, Ph.D., and Stephen R Spindler Ph.D.

"If you started calorie restriction early in life, I think it's possible you might live to be from 140 to 160 years old," says Roy Walford, a pioneer in calorie-restriction research.

Spare but nutritional fare may be one reason that people frequently live to be 120 and older in the Hunza region of the Himalayan Mountains, says Jay Milton Hoffman, Ph.D., who studied the population under the auspices of the National Geriatrics Society. The secret of Hunza longevity, Hoffman believes, is a low-fat, high-fiber vegetarian diet.

"The people of Hunza are not affected by degenerative diseases," he says, "because they do not partake of those things which cause these ailments."

that we pack on pounds. Genes play a role. If your parents or grandparents were big, you may have inherited the tendency. But don't blame the whole spare tire on genes.

Americans simply eat too much. We eat when we're happy. We eat when we're sad. We eat to celebrate special occasions. And Lord knows we love an all-you-can-eat buffet. But what might happen if we went to a buffet—and ate only what our bodies required to stay healthy?

Limiting calories is a sure-fire way to lose weight. But if we carry that concept too far—if we starve ourselves—the opposite occurs. As many as half of all adult Americans are on a diet and nearly two out of every three of us will try to lose weight at least once this year.

But drastically cutting calories, which is how 82 percent of women and 77 percent of men say they try to lose weight, is harmful to your health—and it doesn't work. Dieting failures are as high as 98 percent— and you've got a 73-percent chance of ending up fatter than you were before you started your diet.

That's because low-calorie dieting slows metabolism, the mechanism by which your body burns fat. Your body actually remains in slow mode even after you stop dieting, so you end up storing fat.

Compulsive dieting also can lead to eating disorders, such as bingeing, anorexia nervosa and bulimia. Untreated, eating disorders can cause thyroid problems, malnutrition, anemia, fatigue, ruptured esophagus, rotted teeth, cardiac arrest, multiple organ failure, and strokes.

Do You Have An Eating Disorder?

Eating disorders, including bingeing, anorexia nervosa and bulimia, disrupt the lives of more than 8 million Americans. While eating disorders often are associated with the young, doctors report seeing more middle-aged and elderly patients from all walks of life.

Researchers at New York State Psychiatric Institute studied 200 people who admitted to hours-long eating episodes during which they lost control and ate until they were stuffed. The researchers concluded that the typical binge eater:

—has at least two binge-eating episodes a week during a six-month period.
—eats rapidly, often when not hungry.
—frequently eats alone, at unscheduled times.
—feels disturbed, depressed or guilty about overeating.

Anorexics, on the other hand, severely restrict their food intake, or stop eating altogether. Bulimia compels people to binge and then purge themselves by vomiting or taking laxatives.

Eating disorders are complex illnesses that almost always are accompanied by emotional or psychological problems.

Here are some warning signs to help you know whether you or someone you love should get help. People with eating disorders may:

—be preoccupied with food.
—prefer to eat alone.
—eat what others would consider excessive amounts.
—feel ashamed after overeating.
—lose weight rapidly.
—wear layered clothing to hide their bodies.
—be extremely sensitive to cold temperatures.
—go to the bathroom as soon as they finish eating.
—hide diet pills or laxatives.

How do we lose weight and maintain our health at the same time? By choosing real, wholesome foods and getting sufficient exercise.

> *Eat what you want, but eat a wide variety of foods in moderation. A little bit of everything is better than a lot of one thing.*

The Best Way to Lose
There are a number of strategies you can employ to lose weight successfully and safely. Here are some tips to help you burn fat quickly:

- Eat breakfast. "Always remember that skipping meals leads to binge eating," says dietitian Kathy Stone. As you sleep, your body's metabolism slows down and you burn calories at a reduced rate. Breakfast jump-starts metabolism. Breakfast should be low fat and contain moderate amounts of metabolism-boosting protein, such as skim milk, low-fat cottage cheese, nonfat yogurt or nonfat cream cheese. And if you eat fiber-rich complex carbohydrates, such as whole grains, you're less likely to overeat high-fat foods at lunch.
- Within an hour of rising engage in at least five minutes of physical activity, such as taking a walk or watching the morning news as you pedal a stationary bicycle at a moderate pace.
- Eat snacks to rev up your metabolism. We have a physiological need to eat every two hours or so. Snacks to choose from include whole-grain bagels, low fat muffins, low-fat cookies, fresh fruit or juice, vegetable sticks, or lentil or bean soup.

- Drink ice water. Ice-cold water is a calorie-burning fluid. It requires more than 200 calories of metabolic heat to warm yourself to proper body temperature. "Water may be the simplest, most powerful key to fat loss," says Ellington Darden, Ph.D., an exercise scientist and director of research for Nautilus Sports/Medical Industries. Drinking water also makes you want to eat less. "Drinking generous amounts of water is overwhelmingly the number-one way to head off food cravings and reduce appetite," says George L. Blackburn, M.D., Ph.D., associate professor at Harvard Medical School and director of the Center for the Study of Nutrition Medicine at New England Deaconess Hospital in Boston.
- Limit your intake of caffeinated beverages. These are diuretics and promote loss of fluids, which makes you feel hungrier.
- Cut back on booze. Alcoholic drinks hold empty calories. The body burns fewer fat calories when you drink alcohol, according to a recent Swiss study.
- Take out the fat. "Ninety-seven percent of all fat calories are converted to body fat," reported the late Robert E. T. Stark, M.D., author of *Controlling Fat for Life* and former president of the American Society of Bariatric Physicians. Don't give up your favorite foods, he advises. But cut the fat in them and eat a variety. Emphasize the food tastes you love, but create low-calorie versions.
- Spice up your meals. Foods laced with hot chili pepper and mustard have been shown to help boost the body's metabolic rate and burn more calories.
- Consider supplements. But not those quack diet pills you see on TV (see pages 36-37 and chapter 3, *Supplements*.

Of course no chapter on nutrition would be complete without discussion of the famous—or infamous—**Atkins diet**. In the 1970s Atkins shocked the medical community by recommending that dieters eat all the meat, cheese, eggs and butter they pleased. To lose weight quickly, he said, you have to give up carbohydrates, including bread, rice and pasta.

Could such a diet possibly work? Yes. More doctors, in fact, have begun to rethink their earlier criticisms and now are prescribing the Atkins diet for overweight patients.

Carbo Controversy - The Atkins Diet

It sounds preposterous. Eat meat, cheese and fat to your heart's delight—and still lose weight. But that's exactly what Dr. Robert Atkins recommends in a diet that's been scorned for decades but now is beginning to gain respect from nutritionists.

NUTRITION

"For a large percentage of the population, perhaps 30 to 40 percent, low-fat diets are counterproductive," says Eleftheria Maratos-Flier, director of obesity research at Harvard's Joslin Diabetes Center. "They have the paradoxical effect of making people gain weight."

Atkins has been ridiculed by the medical community since 1972, when he published *Dr. Atkins' Diet Revolution*. The book advises dieters to load up on proteins and fats and cut out most carbohydrates, including breads, pasta and rice.

The American Medical Association branded the Atkins diet a "bizarre regimen." But in the last five years, nutrition researchers have begun to rethink their criticisms. Perhaps, they say, there is some merit to Atkins's methods.

To understand the controversial Atkins diet, we have to step back in time. Before the 1970s, most doctors concurred that carbohydrates were the culprits in the war on obesity. Pass on the pasta, they urged patients; instead, go for lean meats and vegetables, with limited amounts of fat. Fats and proteins, doctors reasoned, left diners feeling full and satisfied, so they were less likely to overeat.

Then along came the fast-food industry that has made the good old U.S.A. famous—or infamous—the world over. Americans in droves gobbled up fatty, cholesterol-packed burgers and greasy, salty fries. And why not? Face it, fast food tastes good. But as we all know, eating a steady diet of junk food is a good way to land yourself in a hospital.

Concerned that heart disease rates would shoot through the national roof, the government reacted. By 1984 the National Institutes of Health was urging Americans over the age of 2 to eat far less fat and far more carbohydrates, such as pasta, rice and potatoes. On the surface, that advice makes sense. Fat is loaded with nine calories per gram; carbs have only four. Ever obedient, Americans complied, or tried to. Before we knew it, shunning fat had become almost a national obsession.

America's food industry jumped on the bandwagon. Hoping to cash in on new dietary guidelines, manufacturers began to suck the fat out of everything. Soon grocery store shelves overflowed with fat-free cookies, fat-free cakes, fat-free chips, fat-free yogurt—fat-free everything.

We couldn't seem to get enough of the new fat-free foods. And why not? If fat makes us fat and manufacturers remove the fat from foods we love, we can eat and eat and eat and not gain weight. Right? Wrong.

As any chef will tell you, fat is a major carrier of flavor. That's why foods laden with fats taste good. To perk up bland fat-free foods, producers added sugar—usually high-fructose corn syrup—and that set the stage for a national health crisis.

The more fat-free foods we consumed, the more calories we packed on—400 more a day, on average, since the government began touting low-fat diets. We're eating far more carbohydrates, too. Since 1970, annual grain consumption has mushroomed by almost 60 pounds per person. No wonder then that nearly one in four Americans now is considered to be obese.

How was that possible, doctors asked, when the percentage of fat in the American diet has been decreasing for two decades? Not only should we be thinner, our rate of heart disease should be substantially lower. But it isn't.

The NIH has spent millions of dollars trying to establish a link between dietary fat and cardiac disease. Five major studies have revealed no such relationship. Indeed, other studies have shown that our bodies require certain fats to function properly. Unsaturated fats, such as olive oil, raise levels of beneficial cholesterol and lower levels of harmful cholesterol. Our brains, moreover, are mostly fat and must have nutrients such as omega-3 fatty acids. Now scientists are coming to the conclusion that some fats are necessary even to maintain proper levels of weight.

As Walter Willet, chairman of the Department of Nutrition at Harvard School of Public Health, says, "The idea that all fat is bad for you may have contributed to the obesity epidemic."

Enter Dr. Atkins. In 1963 the Manhattan cardiologist read about low-carb diets in the *Journal of the American Medical Association* and decided to try one himself. Atkins was amazed to discover that his extra pounds seemed to melt away. He began to look at the effects carbohydrates have on our bodies.

Carbohydrates are dense, starchy foods, such as breads, pasta, rice and potatoes. When we eat such foods, our bodies break down carbohydrates into sugar molecules, which are transported through the bloodstream. Now the pancreas kicks in, secreting insulin to regulate the body's blood-sugar levels. Insulin shunts blood sugar into the muscles and liver so that our bodies can use it as fuel.

Insulin also functions like a switch to regulate the way we metabolize fat. When the switch is on, we burn carbohydrates for energy and store excess calories as fat. When it's off, our bodies burn fat as fuel.

As we gain weight, insulin makes it easier to store fat and harder to lose it. Insulin also affects hunger levels. If insulin lowers your blood sugar, you may find that you are hungry. That's what happens to diabetics. When they get too much insulin, their blood sugar level drops and they crave food. Thus they eat more and insulin stores the calories as fat.

Sugar, starches and anything made from processed flour are considered to be high glycemic-index carbohydrates—that is, they are quickly absorbed in the blood stream and cause a spike in blood sugar, which spurs the pancreas to release a surge of insulin. The insulin stores the blood sugar. A few hours later, levels are lower than before you ate. Your body thinks it has run out of fuel, but your insulin levels are still high enough to prevent you from burning your own fat. The result is hunger. You eat more and gain weight. And the cycle goes on.

Atkins's plan was to help the body to burn its own fat. His high-protein regimen seems to do just that. Nutritionists call the diet ketogenic. If you get your insulin levels down low enough you'll enter a state called ketosis. The muscles and tissues burn body fat for energy in the form of fat molecules produced by the liver called ketones.

That's what happens when people fast or starve. Understandably the idea that dieters were "starving" concerned most doctors, who assailed Atkins as promoting a dangerous regimen. Now, however, they're not so sure.

"Ketosis is a normal physiologic state," says NIH researcher Richard Veech. "Our bodies are supposed to burn fat."

The proof is in the (fat-laden) pudding. Several studies have shown that the Atkins diet seems to work for most people. A study at George Washington University Medical Center in 1980 followed two dozen obese people as they tried the Atkins diet for eight weeks. The participants lost an average of 17 pounds each with no adverse effects.

What's the bottom line? If you have trouble losing weight—and many of us do—the Atkins diet probably will help you to shed pounds. But is the Atkins plan a diet you can follow for life? Probably not, at least without some modifications.

Your body, after all, needs a certain amount of carbohydrates, and remember that not all carbs are bad for you. Moderate servings of whole grains are fine, and beans are the perfect food for diabetics because they release their sugars slowly.

But do go easy on the carbs. Opt for more lean meats and vegetables. And by all means, shun sugary soft drinks, so-called "wet carbs." These are killers. Drink fruit juices instead.

If you'd like to try the Atkins diet, or a modified version, talk with you doctor. Come up with a plan to suit your body and its needs.

From Soup to Nuts

It's clear that food plays an enormous role in attaining and maintaining good health. "We've seen the future—and the future is food," says Mitchell Gaynor, M.D., head of medical oncology at New York's Strang-Cornell Cancer Prevention Center.

Barnard thinks that as our population ages, insurance companies are going to balk at paying for coronary bypasses and other operations. "Instead," he predicts, "they're going to send people through clinical programs to teach them how to adopt healthier lifestyles. They'll learn how to cook vegetarian meals, take a half-hour walk every day, and meditate regularly."

In the meantime, there are several steps you can take to eat a healthier diet, says Arnold Fox, M.D., an anti-aging expert in Beverly Hills, California:

• Think of your diet as a pyramid. The widest part of the pyramid is made up of fresh vegetables, fruits, and whole grains. On top of that, add smaller amounts of fish, low-fat dairy products, lean poultry, nuts, and seeds. At the top of the pyramid are the snack foods and deserts. Eat only tiny amounts of these.
• Keep your sugar consumption low. Nature has already packed inside its foods as much sugar as you need. "A little added sugar won't harm most of us," Fox says, "but a lot will hurt many of us."
• Don't add salt to your foods. Excess salt has a number of bad effects, and nature has already put plenty of salt in food.
• Keep fat consumption within healthful limits. Go easy on snack foods, processed foods, and other foods with added fats. Eat more healthy fats, such as olive oil.
• Eat slowly. Enjoy your food. Give your appetite center time to tell you that you've had enough, before you've had too much. If you're not hungry, don't eat. "Let your stomach guide you, not the clock."
• Drink plenty of water, at least six to eight, eight-ounce glasses a day.

Above all, enjoy your food. Take a tip from Europeans, who turn dinners into social affairs that celebrate family, friends and fine living.

Supplement Savvy

There are hundreds of diet supplements on the market and all of them claim to help you lose weight effortlessly. Do they work? No. The only way to drop pounds and keep them off is to choose healthy foods, limit portion size and exercise. But some studies suggest that two supplements may improve your odds:

Aspirin. Recent studies suggest that aspirin helps to rev up your metabolism, spurring your body to burn off fat before it has a chance to turn your thighs flabby or wrap itself into a spare tire around your waist.

"A low dose of aspirin—about one tablet—can speed up loss of body fat by promoting thermogensis," says author and nutritional expert Robert Haas, Ph.D.

Thermogenesis is the chemical process by which your body generates heat. It is that heat that burns calories to produce energy instead of storing them as fat. The problem is that not everyone burns calories efficiently.

Dean Brenner, M.D., associate professor of internal medicine and pharmacology at the University of Michigan Medical Center gave 15 test subjects an aspirin a day for two weeks. Tests later showed that aspirin had stopped fat from accumulating in the subjects' bodies.

How does aspirin accomplish this miracle? Scientists don't know for sure. One theory is that aspirin interferes with production of prostaglandins, fatty acids involved with pain that also help to regulate your internal furnace.

Taking too much aspirin, on the other hand, can thin your blood to dangerous levels and damage the lining of your stomach.

Chitosan. Studies from Norway, Japan and Texas A&M University have concluded that chitosan is an effective fat blocker. Made from the exoskeletons of shellfish, chitosan acts like a fat magnet. "If you eat an occasional candy bar and take chitosan, it will absorb three to six times its weight in fat, flushing it out of your system," says Brenda Adderly, author of the *Complete Guide to Nutritional Supplements.*

Chitosan also reduces unhealthy cholesterol while raising levels of beneficial cholesterol. And, because of its cleansing properties, the supplement may protect against colon cancer.

The down side is that you might be tempted to use chitosan as a remedy for overeating. "It's really for people who already adhere to a good diet and exercise program, and don't have severe eating disorders," says Adderly. Although it's unlikely, chitosan could cause problems if you are allergic to shellfish.

Take at least one gram before or with lunch or dinner. Drink at last one eight-ounce glass of water with each tablet or you may get constipated. Drink water throughout the day so the fiber doesn't get backed up.

Endnote: Food Pharmacy

For many people suffering from a variety of common ailments, a change in diets may produce favorable results. Here are some common foods and the painful conditions they may alleviate:

Fruits
Avocados: carpal tunnel syndrome
Bananas: digestion, carpal tunnel syndrome
Blueberries, cherries, dried currants, dried dates, prunes, raspberries, apples (notably, Granny Smith), oranges and persimmons: blunt pain; they're high in salicylates, natural chemicals that act like aspirin:
Figs: psoriasis
Papayas: digestion

Peaches: arthritis
Pineapples: digestion, inflammation

Vegetables
Broccoli: carpal tunnel syndrome
Brussels sprouts: carpal tunnel syndrome
Cabbage: ulcers
Chickpeas: carpal tunnel syndrome
Collard greens: menstrual pain, osteoporosis
Legumes: carpal tunnel syndrome, diabetes
Onions: respiratory conditions
Peas: arthritis
Peppers (sweet and hot): contain aspirin-like chemicals that can blunt pain
Plantains: ulcers
Potatoes: headaches, menstrual pain, carpal tunnel syndrome, fibromyalgia
Shitake mushrooms: respiratory problems
Soy beans (and soy products): menstrual pain, carpal tunnel syndrome, gall stones
Spinach: carpal tunnel syndrome, depression
Sweet potatoes: carpal tunnel syndrome
Yucca: arthritis

Grains
Bread: menstrual pain, depression
Cereal: diarrhea, depression
Crackers: headaches
Oats: menstrual pain
Pasta: menstrual pain, depression
Rice: digestion, headaches, menstrual pain
Whole grains (all): diabetes, fibromyalgia

Nuts and Seeds
Almonds: they're high in aspirin-like chemicals that can blunt pain
Brazil nuts: depression
Sunflower seeds: depression

Dairy
Yogurt: diarrhea, menstrual pain, respiratory pain
Milk: osteoporosis, menstrual pain

Poultry
Chicken liver: depression
Chicken (soup): respiratory problems

Fish
Fatty fishes (tuna, salmon, etc.): arthritis, menstrual pain
Seafood (tuna, oysters, clams, swordfish): depression

Oils
Anti-inflammatory oils (black current, borage, evening primrose flaxseed, hemp, linseed, canola, soy, walnut, wheat germ): arthritis
Heart-healthy oils (olive, etc.): menstrual pain

Beverages
Alcohol (small quantities): ulcers, menstrual pain, gallstones
Coffee: migraines, menstrual pain, depression, kidney stones
Cranberry juice: urinary pain
Green tea: arthritis, ulcers, kidney stones
Water: urinary pain, kidney stones

Nutrition Action Plan

•**Take stock.** Keep a food journal for a week. Note what you eat and when—then ask yourself why? Are you hungry—or are you eating because youíre stressed out?

•**Go for the garlic.** Adding garlic to your diet is one of the easiest ways to protect yourself from heart disease and build up your immune system. Whatís more, garlic enhances the flavor of just about every dish. Serious garlic lovers, in fact, have been known to add it to ice cream!

•**Cut back on carbs.** No need to swear off potatoes, pasta and pastries—but nobody needs as much as most of us consume.

•**Crunch a cruciferous vegetable.** Have at least one serving a week of cabbage, broccoli or cauliflower. They contain cancer-fighting chemicals—and they taste good, too!

•**Pour on the olive oil.** Each time you reach for butter or margarine, substitute a fruity splash of heart-healthy liquid gold.

2. Herbs

Get Your Medicine From Mother Nature's Pharmacy

Herbs are our original medicines. People have been using them for centuries to prevent and treat a number of illnesses. You may find it beneficial to add herbs to your health regimen, too.

Next time a flu bug knocks you for a loop, don't turn to the bathroom medicine chest for relief—head for the kitchen.

"The kitchen spice shelf is a convenient place to discover the medicinal value of herbs," says herbalist Michael Tierra, author of *The Way of Herbs.* "The common culinary herbs and spices so often added to foods for flavor also have considerable medicinal use—and they're a safe and natural alternative to the synthetic drugs found in the medicine cabinet."

> *Supplementing your diet with herbs is a great way to get healthy and stay healthy.*

Plants have provided us with many of our most common prescription drugs. Twenty-five percent of medical drugs we use in this country, in fact, come from herbs and other plants that grow in tropical rain forests. Such plants are equipped to fight diseases because they typically contain strong chemicals to fight off jungle predators.

"The aromatic oils that give spices their flavor are chemicals that make up the defense mechanisms that plants use to protect themselves from insects, fungi and bacteria," explains herbalist Michael Castleman, author of *The Healing Herbs.* " All of the oils in spices are antibacterial and antifungal. Thus, they can help us to fight off the germs that make us sick."

Amazing Amazon

Like Sean Connery in the movie *Medicine Man*, David Kingston is searching the Amazon jungles of Suriname for a cancer cure.

"We have not found a drug yet," says Kingston, a chemistry professor at Virginia Polytechnic Institute and State University in Blacksburg, "but we have isolated 25 new chemical entities, and all have biological activity."

The Amazon is packed with plants that may hold cures for cancer, AIDS and other illnesses. Others may contain chemical compounds that could slow the aging process and extend our lives. Some of the most potent Amazon medicines we have today include:

Vincristine. Extracted from a species of periwinkle that grows in the rain forests of Madagascar, this drug has dramatically increased survival from childhood leukemia. Thanks to vincristine, eight out of 10 children stricken with the devastating disease recover fully.

Quinine. For decades this medicine made from South American cinchona bark has been used to save millions around the world from perishing from malaria.

Curare. South American Indians dip their arrowheads in this plant-derived poison. But curare has far more valuable uses. It yields d-turbocurarine and other alkaloids used to treat multiple sclerosis and Parkinson's disease, and it's an essential ingredient of anesthesia.

Those miracle medicines are just a fraction of the healing drugs that may be hidden in the forest. As many as 300 new life-saving drugs—valued at $147 billion—await discovery, according to estimates by Yale economist Robert Mendelsohn and Michael J. Balick, director of the Institute of Economic Botany at the New York Botanical Gardens.

For generations, Indians living in the rain forest have relied on healing plants to cure all sorts of illnesses. From mankind's earliest days, in fact, we have prized herbs for their culinary and healing properties.

"Our ancestors discovered many healing herbs simply by trial and error," Castleman explains. "We'll never know how many roots the ancient Indians dug up before they discovered ginger more than 4,000 years ago."

It wasn't long before early cooks discovered that herbs not only perked up the flavor of foods but imparted healthful benefits.

As far back as 3,000 B.C., Sumerian physicians were chiseling prescriptions for garlic on clay tablets. Egyptians entombed their pharaohs with coriander seeds, and more than 5,000 years ago Ayurvedic healers in India used scores of herbs to treat a multitude of ailments. It was around this time that emperor-sage Shen Nung compiled the first great Chinese herbal, *Pen Tsao Ching* (The Classic of Herbs).

Knowledge of herbal medicines flourished in ancient Greece. Hippocrates, the "father" of western medicine, taught his students how to use herbs to ease pain and cure disease. By the first century A.D., the physician Dioscorides had listed the medicinal properties of more than 500 plants and herbs in the *Materia Medica*, which became the standard medical text used by European physicians for hundreds of years.

In the next century Roman physician Galen wrote medical books that were used throughout Europe for the next 1,500 years. As Roman soldiers spread throughout Europe, they brought their knowledge of herbs to the lands they conquered and also learned more about herbal lore from the people living there. The Romans introduced more than 200 herbs to conquered Britain, including fennel, sage, borage, betony, parsley, rosemary and thyme. Eventually European monks developed "physick" gardens of herbs to heal and monasteries became Europe's learning centers for medicine.

Herbal knowledge continued to evolve. In 1551 William Turner published his *New Herball,* which described 238 British plants. In 1653 Nicholas Culpepper, physician, published an herbal text still in use today.

In the New World, where Native Americans had been using herbs for millennia, colonists brought cuttings and roots of their favorite plants. Herbal lore flourished in America, peaking in the 18th century. The Shakers, members of a Spartan religious sect, became America's first professional herbalists, growing and selling medicinal herbs on a large scale.

Herb use declined after the advent of chemical pharmaceuticals in the 20th century. Beginning in the 1960s and 1970s, however, consumers began to show renewed interest in natural therapies. In the early part of the 21st century, sales of herbal medicines are at an all-time high.

Today, says Castleman, "Scientists are taking a new look at a whole gamut of ancient healing remedies," including many found in our kitchens. Researchers around the world have conducted thousands of studies on the medical efficacy of scores of herbs.

"The problem," Castleman says, "is that the vast majority have been done in Europe or India. That's because in this country, the majority of medical research into new drugs is funded by the pharmaceutical industry. You can't patent herbs, so pharmaceutical companies are not interested in studying them. Nobody's going to spend $10 million to prove that garlic lowers cholesterol because no one could recoup that investment."

Nonetheless, many foreign studies have proved to be reliable, pharmacy professor Varro Tyler, Ph.D., said in an interview before his death in 2001. "Remember that these herbs have been used for centuries, so any serious problems with them have long ago been identified."

Annual sales of herbs and herbal products continue to rise. A third of American adults, in fact, report that they have used herbs medicinally.

"People are beginning to realize that western pharmacological medicine doesn't have all the answers," Castleman says. "They're yearning for a connection with more traditional therapies."

Unlike many prescription and over-the-counter medicines, most herbs produce no harmful side effects, says James Duke, Ph.D., a former U.S. Dept. of Agriculture botanist and author of *The Green Pharmacy*. "Used in moderation," Duke says, "most herbs are more than safe."

Herbs are easy to use. For most kitchen remedies, teas are easiest to prepare. Steep 1 tsp. herb in 1 cup hot water; drink up to 3 cups a day. If you opt to buy capsules or tinctures (herb-infused liquids) from a health-food store or pharmacy, follow directions on the bottle. Remember, check with your doctor before taking any herb, supplement or drug.

Kitchen Cabinet Cures

These days you'll find herbs everywhere – in health-food stores, pharmacies, even doctors' offices. A great place to start making herbal medicines is right in your kitchen.

"All of the herbs that people have in their spice racks have medicinal purposes," Castleman says. "You can use kitchen herbs and spices to treat problems ranging from diarrhea and headache to sore throats and influenza. And in minor emergencies, kitchen staples provide easy-to-reach-for first-aid remedies."

Here are just a few of the kitchen medicines you may want to pull from your spice rack:

Basil. Researchers in Israel say that basil, along with cumin and turmeric, may fight certain cancers, especially of the bladder and prostate. In addition, basil contains chemicals that boost the immune system's ability to function.

Caraway. In some German restaurants you'll be given caraway seeds to chew after packing in a hearty meal. That's because caraway contains two chemicals—carvol and carvene—that soothe the muscles lining the digestive tract. For centuries the herb has been used to relieve indigestion and prevent gas. It's not surprising then that caraway seeds flavor rye bread. In addition, caraway's calming compounds relax uterine muscles, so munching on a handful of seeds may help to ease the pain of menstrual cramps.

Cayenne. Cayenne contains a pain-relieving chemical called capsaicin. So effective is capsaicin at blunting pain that it's an ingredient in many over-the-counter and prescription ointments. Capsaicin appears to work by interfering with the action of Substance P, a chemical in the peripheral nerves that sends pain messages to the brain. Blend cayenne with olive oil and rub on toothaches and arthritic joints. And it may surprise you to learn that you can brew up an indigestion-relieving tea from spicy cayenne. Capsaicin aids digestion by stimulating flow of saliva and stomach secretions. In addition, numerous studies indicate that it kills bacteria; relieves diarrhea; reduces the pain of cluster headaches; and lowers cholesterol levels.

Cinnamon. There is some scientific evidence that cinnamon triples the ability of insulin to metabolize glucose, making it a good spice for diabetics. In addition, cinnamon is strongly antibacterial. That's why it's often used to flavor mouthwashes. As Castleman says, "The oils in cinnamon help to kill the bacteria in the gum line that cause gum disease and tooth decay."

Clove. Grandma was right. You can kill the pain of an aching tooth by swabbing it with clove oil. Researchers attribute the remedy's effectiveness to eugenol, a pain-relieving chemical found abundantly in cloves. In addition, the stimulating aromatic buds increase circulation, improve digestion, prevent gas, and ease symptoms of nausea. Other kitchen herbs containing eugenol include cinnamon and tarragon.

Garlic. At the first sign of a cold or flu, pop a garlic clove or two. You may not be the most popular person in your house, but you'll feel a lot better. One medium-size garlic clove packs the antibacterial punch of about 100,000 units of penicillin. "Garlic is a powerful antibiotic," Castleman says.

The herb's primary constituent is a chemical called alliin. Alliin interacts with an enzyme called allinase, which then transforms into allicin, which kills dozens of harmful bacteria, including those that cause tuberculosis, food poisoning and bladder infections.

When allicin joins forces with ajoene, another of garlic's chemicals, it prevents platelets from forming blood clots that could lead to heart attacks and strokes. In addition, garlic keeps blood vessels elastic. Every time your heart beats, your blood vessels need to expand. Garlic helps them to do that. Thus, garlic is a good natural medicine for preventing and treating heart disease and strokes. Several studies, moreover, conclude that garlic reduces blood pressure and blood sugar levels and may help to prevent and treat cancer, AIDS and other serious diseases.

For medicinal purposes, it's best to eat garlic raw in salads. But there are some good supplements on the market, according to Tyler. "You can derive substantial medical benefits by taking garlic tablets that have been coated so that allicin is protected and released into the small intestine."

Ginger. Did your mother give you ginger ale when you had an upset tummy? If so, her instincts were medically sound. "Ginger is a great stomach soother," says Castleman. "Ginger ale originally was a medicine used to treat indigestion."

Ginger contains chemicals that calm stomach spasms and break down proteins, like digestive enzymes. And for nausea and dizziness caused by motion sickness, ginger works better than Dramamine, according to a study published in the British medical journal *Lancet.* A mug of ginger tea will warm you up if influenza leaves you shivering. And Chinese researchers report that ginger compounds attack the viruses that cause flu.

Ginger also contains chemicals that reduce inflammation, says bestselling author Jason Theodosakis, M.D. "Thus, many people have used ginger to ease the pain of arthritis."

Indian scientists theorize that ginger increases the immune system's ability to fight infections. Because ginger improves circulation, it's a heart-healthy herb. And studies are underway to assess ginger's abilities to shrink cancerous tumors.

Mint. There's nothing better to open up a stuffy nose than a cup of mint tea. Peppermint oil contains menthol, the decongestant chemical found in many over-the-counter cold rubs and nasal sprays. Menthol also calms the muscles in your stomach. That's why many restaurants offer peppermints at the end of a meal. If you're out of peppermint, spearmint works as well. It contains a chemical called carvone, with properties similar to menthol's.

Parsley. Sweeten garlic breath by munching on parsley, which contains high levels of chlorophyll, the active ingredient of many commercial breath fresheners.

The herb is rich in apiol and myristicin, chemicals with significant diuretic properties. German physicians, in fact, prescribe parsley seed tea to reduce fluid buildup in people with high blood pressure. Parsley also may help if you suffer from hay fever or hives. A study in the *Journal of Allergy and Clinical Immunology* finds that parsley inhibits secretion of histamine, a chemical in your body that triggers allergic reactions. And psoralen, another of parsley's chemicals, shows promise in the laboratory for treating some types of cancer. In addition, parsley contains trace elements, including copper, magnesium, molybdenum and zinc.

Pepper. Black pepper, jalapeno peppers, mustard and hot red peppers increase metabolism and may lower risk of certain cancers.

Rosemary. Sidelined by a headache? Nix the ibuprofen and try a cup of rosemary tea. Researchers say this antioxidant herb increases blood flow to the brain. Perhaps that's why ancient Greeks considered rosemary to be a memory booster. What's more, rosemary is high in easy-to-assimilate calcium, which can help to prevent osteoporosis. Follicle-nourishing compounds in the herb make rosemary a great rinse for damaged or dandruff-ridden hair.

Sage. Don't save the sage to spice up your Thanksgiving turkey. Gargle with sage tea the next time your throat's on fire. Studies show that antioxidant sage contains infection-fighting chemicals, and it's high in astringent tannins, which help to heal bleeding gums and mouth ulcers. Sage also has been used to treat diarrhea; excessive perspiration; sinus congestion and inflammation. A study from Germany found that sage reduces blood sugar levels, which means it could help diabetics.

Thyme. When you can't halt the hacking, it's time for a cup of thyme. The herb contains thymol, a chemical that loosens phlegm. Also found in oregano, thymol is a prime ingredient in many commercial cough syrups. In addition, thyme contains carvacol, which relaxes the gastrointestinal tract. Thyme is good for treating bronchitis and other respiratory ailments. It's also been used to relieve laryngitis; diarrhea; chronic gastritis; and lack of appetite. Because of its antiseptic properties, thyme tea makes an excellent mouthwash. Use it as well to treat fungal athlete's foot and to kill skin parasites, including lice.

Turmeric. If you're into Indian food, you know about turmeric, the herb that gives curries their yellow color. Like ginger, turmeric increases circulation, which helps to prevent and treat heart disease. And, says, Castleman, "Turmeric is a powerful antibiotic that kills microbes."

Turmeric and other plant foods (including soy, rosemary, carrots and grapes) also contain compounds known as Cox-2 inhibitors, which impede the growth of new blood vessels and may be helpful for treating tumors.

Garden Magic

Medicinal herbs aren't confined to the spice rack. Step outside the kitchen door and you'll discover myriad health benefits from herbs that may be growing in your back yard.

Aloe Vera. This common houseplant is a wonderful remedy for minor burns and cuts. "Chemicals in aloe stimulate growth of new skin cells, helping healthy new tissue to form," says Castleman. Simply break off a leaf, squeeze out the gelatinous material and rub it on the wound.

HERBS

Echinacea. Also known as purple coneflower, echinacea is the number-one best-selling herb in the United States. Take it at the first sign of a cold. Several studies show that echinacea boosts the immune system's ability to ward off illnesses. According to Tyler: "It can cut the duration of a cold by several days."

There are three different species of echinacea on the market, and some of these are used interchangeably. Studies show that the juice extracted from the flowers and leaves of a species called *echinacea purpurea* are most effective. The problem in this country is that when you buy echinacea you don't always know what you're getting.

Ginkgo. Ginkgo may not make you smarter, but several studies indicate that this ancient Asian herb does improve cerebral function, and may prove to be a valuable natural remedy for treating the symptoms of Alzheimer's Disease, a devastating illness that erases the memory and personality of its victims.

The U.S. Food and Drug Administration does not recognize *ginkgo biloba* as a medicine. But, "research on ginkgo and Alzheimer's is producing extremely good results in France and Germany," says herb researcher Daniel B. Mowrey, Ph.D.

Indeed, Europeans have been using ginkgo extract for years to fight off Alzheimer's and other cerebral disorders associated with aging, including forgetfulness; mild confusion; tinnitus, or ringing in the ears; and inability to concentrate. In some countries, in fact, ginkgo is a registered drug, among the most commonly prescribed for treating organic brain disorders.

Ginkgo's benefits seem to derive from its ability to improve circulation in virtually every area of the body, especially the brain. Ginkgo opens up blood vessels and keeps them supple, thus helping to prevent circulatory problems. By improving blood flow, ginkgo enhances the body's ability to nourish itself.

Ginkgo also helps to fight free radicals, those highly reactive molecules that are absorbed in our body when we breath polluted air or eat harmful foods such as fats. Free radicals contribute to many diseases. Researchers think they probably play a role in degenerative diseases, such as cancer and Alzheimer's, and in the aging process itself. Antioxidants such as ginkgo scavenge free radicals, reacting with them and leaving harmless molecules in their place.

Ginkgo moreover has the ability to interfere with a bodily substance called platelet activation factor (PAF). Discovered in 1972, PAF is involved in a staggering number of biological procedures, including asthma attacks, organ graft rejection, arterial blood flow, and formation of internal blood clots that can lead to heart attacks and strokes. By inhibiting PAF, ginkgo may keep us from developing many of the diseases that strike as we grow older.

One of the most famous ginkgo studies of aging-induced cerebral disorders was reported in 1986 by the French medical journal *La Presse Medicale*. Researchers developed a scale of 17 items to evaluate 166 geriatric patients in several centers. Markers included vivacity, short-term memory, disturbances in orientation, anxiety, depression, emotional stability, initiative, cooperation, sociability, personal care, ability to walk, appetite, vertigo, fatigue, headache, sleep and ringing in ears. After taking ginkgo extract for three months, the subjects improved in every area, and they continued to improve over time.

St. John's Wort. In recent years Americans by the droves took this herb to treat depression. The question is, does it work? "It does work for mild to moderate depression in many people," according to Tyler.

St. John's wort can take several weeks before you notice its effects. "Herbs are gentle medicines," Tyler says. "They don't work immediately, but instead work slowly over a long period of time.

There have been some reports that St. John's wort causes extreme sensitivity to sunlight. Tyler says, however, that the condition is rare. "If you take the standard dosage – up to 900 mg a day of St. John's wort – you should be fine."

An Herb for Women

An herb called **chasteberry** is helping many women to deal with symptoms of menopause.

"Many of the women I see in my practice use chasteberry to ease a number of symptoms associated with reproductive health," says Arnold Fox, M.D., a California cardiologist and pain expert. "Most of them say that chasteberry helps them a great deal."

Chasteberry's constituents include monoterpenes, such as aguside, eurostosie, and aucubin, as well as the flavonoids casticin, chryso-splenol and vitexin. The herb's progesterone-like effect appears to derive from its volatile oils.

Preliminary research indicates that chasteberry's chemical compounds are able to adjust the production of certain female hormones. German tests of laboratory animals, for example, have discovered that chasteberry stimulates release of a chemical called Leutenizing Hormone (LH), and inhibits the release of Follicle Stimulating Hormone (FSH).

These hormone-regulating chemicals appear to quell pain. At a clinic in London, researcher Alan Stewart gave 30 women with premenstrual symptoms 1.5 g a day of dried chasteberry in capsule form. Stewart found that the women reported a 60 percent reduction in symptoms such as anxiety, nervous tension, insomnia and mood changes.

Chasteberry also has been used effectively to treat many of the symptoms associated with menopause. Sometimes the herb is used alone, and sometimes it is combined with other herbs that nourish the female glandular system. These include angelica, licorice root and black cohosh. Combinations of chasteberry, motherwort and wild yam may help to calm the rapid heartbeat that often accompanies hot flashes.

An Herb for Men

Most men over the age of 60—and many over 50—develop some symptoms associated with benign prostatic hyperplasia, also known as enlarged prostate. Now more men are preventing and treating the condition with an extract made from the berries of the common **saw palmetto plant**.

Saw palmetto is a shrub that grows profusely in the southeastern part of the United States. The medicine comes from an extract of saw palmetto berries. Several studies have shown that this extract is quite effective at shrinking enlarged prostate glands—and it's far less expensive than many pharmaceutical medicines prescribed by doctors.

"Studies have shown that saw palmetto can improve urinary flow rates and reduce symptoms like urinary hesitancy and weak flow," says Alan R. Gaby, M.D., former president of the American Holistic Medical Association. "In many cases it works as well or better than prescription drugs—and it's cheaper and safer."

Studies in Europe indicate that an extract from saw palmetto berries appears to counteract the effects of male sex hormones, called androgens, that may cause prostate enlargement." reported the late pharmacy expert Varro Tyler.

In Belgium researchers gave saw palmetto extract to 505 men with benign prostate disease. At the end of the trial, the researchers concluded that saw palmetto had aided urinary flow, reduced residual urinary volume and prostate size, and otherwise improved the patients' quality of life. Saw palmetto, moreover, began to produce results within 45 days. After 90 days of saw palmetto treatment, 88 percent of patients and their physicians said they considered the therapy to be effective.

Some physicians say there is sufficient clinical evidence that saw palmetto works better than many prescription medications to reduce enlarged prostates. "The fat-soluble extract of saw palmetto berries is much effective than Proscar, and saw palmetto costs one fourth the cost of Proscar," says Julian Whitaker, M.D., founder and director of The Whitaker Wellness Institute Inc. in Newport Beach, Calif.

Moreover, Whitaker says, "Proscar is effective in less than 50 percent of cases after patients have taken it for a full year. Saw palmetto extract effective in nearly 90 percent of patients, usually after four to six weeks."

What's in Store?

Used for centuries, herbal medicine fell into disrepair after the advent of pharmaceutical drugs in the mid-20th century. Today, as consumers seek more ways to live natural lives, herbal medicine seems to be more popular than ever. Some experts are even predicting that herbal medicine once again will be a mainstream treatment option.

"I think it will become integrated into conventional medicine," says Tyler. "Physicians will begin to prescribe herbal products along with pharmaceutical medicines."

It's true that more conventional doctors are learning about the healing properties of herbs. They have to—so many of their patients have begun asking for herbal remedies.

"People today are more serious about taking care of their own health," says Tyler. "They're tired of the impersonal, expensive nature of modern medicine."

Herbs, on the other hand are relatively inexpensive. They work in many cases and most important of all, they have few side effects.

Consider adding herbs to your new regimen for a healthy lifestyle.

Fix it with Herbs!

Head to the kitchen cabinet, and not the medicine cabinet, for daily protection against both big and small problems. Or to your own garden, even if it's a small indoor pot of herbs you've grown yourself. Next time you experience one of the following ailments, try one of these cures:

Bladder or Prostrate Problems – use more basil, cumin or turmeric in your recipes, or take some Saw palmetto extract for prostrate concerns

Indigestion – try munching on caraway seeds, eat some ginger, or brew a tea from spicy cayenne

Toothache – swab it with clove oil, or blend cayenne with olive oil and rub on teeth

Arthritic joints – try the olive oil/cayenne blend above

Cold or Flu – pop a few garlic cloves, drink some mint tea, or squeeze the juice out of the echinacea flower from your herb garden

Headache – drink a cup of rosemary tea

Bad Breath – munch on some parsley

Sore Throat – gargle with sage

Cough – drink some thyme tea

Minor Burns or Cuts – rub some aloe vera on it

Endnote: More Healthy Herbs

Black Cohosh
Cimifuga racemosa
Treats menstrual conditions, including premenstrual syndrome and menopause; also has been used to manage prostate cancer, lower blood pressure and treat arthritis.

Chamomile
Matriara recutita, M. chamomilla, Chamomilla recutita, Anthemis nobilis
Treats digestive disorders, spasms, stomach upset, inflammation, irritations and infections of the mouth and gums

Feverfew
Chrysanthemum parthenium
Use to prevent and treat migraine headaches; may help rheumatoid arthritis and other inflammatory disorders.

Ginseng
Panax ginseng
Rejuvenates all systems of body; promotes sexual function.

Goldenseal
Hydrastis canadensis
Works as an antibiotic; immune stimulant.

Hawthorn
Crataegus oxyacantha
Heart tonic; lowers blood pressure, reduces chest pain, treats tachycardia, controls athersclerosis.

Horehound
Marrubium vulgare
Treats coughs, especially those that require an expectorant; has been used as a remedy for colds, flu and fevers.

Kava Kava
Piper methysticum
Relieves stress; promotes feelings of well-being.

Lemon Balm
Melissa officinalis
Promotes relaxation, aids digestion, treats wounds and viral infections.

Licorice
Glycyrrhiza glabra
Treats coughs, ulcers, arthritis, herpes, hepatitis and cirrhosis.

Milk Thistle
Silybum marianum
Good for liver diseases, including cirrhosis and hepatitis, counteracts effects of some toxins.

Slippery Elm
Ulmus rubra, U. fulva
Treats wounds, coughs, sore throat, digestive complaints.

Valerian
Valeriana officinalis
Relieves stress, promotes sleep.

White Willow
Salix alba
Contains aspirinlike chemicals; reduces fevers, kills pain, fights inflammation, treats menstrual cramps.

Herbs Action Plan

•**Spice it up.** Experiment with herbs and spices. Try a new seasoning with every meal. Smell it, taste it. Soon you'll be adding healthy herbs and spices to everything you cook.

•**Treat yourself.** Discuss disease-specific herbs with your doctor. Some studies indicate that hawthorn is beneficial for heart conditions; others show that feverfew is effective for preventing and treating migraine headaches. Most common herbs, in fact, have been used as medicines for centuries.

•**Plant an herb garden.** Herbs are among the easiest of plants to grow. It's practically impossible to kill them. Having pots near your kitchen will make it easier for you to incorporate herbs in your diet.

•**Take time for tea.** Get in the habit of brewing a comforting cup of herbal tea in the evening. Try a relaxing herb, such as chamomile, to help you sleep.

•**Power up.** The first time you sneeze, pop a couple of echinacea capsules. Echinacea boosts your immune system, enabling your body to ward off colds and other minor ailments.

3. Supplements

Give Your Health a Boost

It's true. We cannot live by bread alone. Talk with your doctor about adding vitamins, minerals and other natural supplements to your diet of healthy foods.

Eating right can save your life. But you can't obtain all of your life-extending nutrients from food alone.

Tomatoes, for example, are a great source of lycopene, a natural chemical that appears to fight prostate cancer. But you'd have to eat six pounds of tomatoes a day to get all of the lycopene you need, says Omer Kucuk, M.D., who has studied the supplement at Karmanos Cancer Institute in Detroit.

Even the healthiest eaters need supplements. That's because as we age, our bodies begin to slow production of key enzymes, hormones and compounds we need to function at our best. "And most Americans consume a diet that is inadequate in nutritional value," says Julian Whitaker, M.D., founder and director of The Whitaker Wellness Institute Inc. in Newport Beach, California.

Fortunately, you can provide your body with the nutrients its needs by adding natural supplements to your diet, says William Faloon, vice president of the Life Extension Foundation, a company in Fort Lauderdale, Florida, that researches and sells supplements.

"If you think of the body as an automobile's combustion engine and supplements as spark plugs, you have a fairly good idea of how these amazing substances work for us," says pharmacist and author Earl Mindell, Ph.D.

Aspirin is more than a pain reliever. It's one of the first supplements you should add to your daily regimen.

What's more, there's nothing mysterious or magical about supplements. Look in your medicine cabinet and you'll find that you probably already have a number of supplements that can help you in your quest for a healthy lifestyle.

What Are Supplements?

Supplements include vitamins, minerals, hormones and other natural substances. Once confined to shelves of health-food stores, supplements are showing up everywhere these days, from supermarkets and pharmacies to department stores.

"The pharmaceutical industry has pumped out hundreds of different medicines," says Arnold Fox, M.D., who often recommends supplements

Not Just for Headaches

After it was discovered in the 19th century, aspirin was hailed as a miracle drug. Today scientists conclude that this common pain reliever may indeed save your life.

Numerous studies show that low-dose aspirin—about 80 milligrams a day—may reduce risk of a heart attack by 40 percent and cut stroke risk by 18 percent. More than 50 clinical studies document the safety and efficacy of aspirin as a cardiovascular drug. In fact, the American College of Chest Physicians recommends aspirin for all people over 50 who have at least one risk factor for heart disease and no conditions (such as an ulcer) that make aspirin consumption inadvisable.

Taking aspirin regularly also could halve your chances of developing colon cancer and lower the likelihood of having a migraine attack by 20 percent. Scientists in Baltimore theorize that aspirin may increase brain circulation and reduce inflammation associated with dementia and other forms of cognitive decline associated with Alzheimer's disease. In addition, several studies indicate that aspirin reduces blood levels of C-reactive protein, which inflames the inside of arterial walls and may cause acute blockage in a coronary or cerebral artery. Aspirin also makes blood platelets less likely to clump and form life-threatening blood clots.

to his patients in Los Angeles. "More people now are looking for a natural alternative."

A good multivitamin a day really can go a long way toward getting you healthy and keeping you that way. That may be why more than 100 million Americans take a vitamin each morning.

Take Your Vitamins

Vitamins are organic chemicals that act as catalysts. Each vitamin has a function, from helping bone growth and maintaining healthy skin to assisting cells in processing energy. If your body falls short in one vitamin, any number of vital functions that depend on that vitamin are compromised.

Nutritionists divide the 13 essential vitamins into two groups based on their behavior in the body. Water-soluble vitamins—C and the eight B vitamins—are short-lived, fast-acting compounds stored in the watery parts of body cells, but not for long. The body quickly puts these vitamins to work assisting cells in chemical reactions and energy processing, and excretes any excess vitamins.

Fat-soluble vitamins—A, D, E and K—are found in fatty parts of cells and regulate a wide variety of metabolic processes. These vitamins tend to be put into long-term storage and then are drawn upon as the body needs them.

Heart Healthy

Vitamins may help to heal your heart. *The Journal of the American Medical Association* recently reported that a six-month regimen of folic acid, vitamin B12 and vitamin B6 helped to prevent recurrence of blocked arteries in patients who had undergone coronary angioplasty.

The treatment works by lowering levels of homocysteine, an amino acid that appears to trigger heart attacks, according to Dr. Guido Schnyder, assistant professor in the cardiology division at the University of California at San Diego.

Dr. Robert Bonow, chief of cardiology at Northwestern Memorial Hospital in Chicago and president of the American Heart Association, said the study offers more evidence that B vitamins are important in maintaining healthy blood vessels.

Several vitamins have been singled out for their ability to slow down or even prevent the onset of age-related diseases, such as heart disease and cancer. Some vitamins may even potentially slow the aging process itself. Chief among these are antioxidants. These supplements fight so-called free radicals. Free radicals are not counterculture activists who have been in hiding for the last 30 years. They're oxygen molecules gone haywire and they appear to contribute to many disease processes.

> *Antioxidants are among the most important supplements you can take.*

Put the Brake on Free Radicals

You've probably heard a lot about free radicals and supplements used to eradicate them. But what are free radicals?

To get the energy they need, our body cells use oxygen to burn fuels such as glucose, or blood sugar. In the process, some oxygen molecules may lose an electron. Such molecules now are known as free radicals, and they attempt to replace lost electrons by raiding other molecules that make up the cell. As it steals an electron, the free radical oxygen molecule transforms the unsuspecting molecule into a new free radical.

"Soon a chain reaction of electron theft begins that can produce widespread damage to the chemistry and function of the cell," says Denham Harmon, M.D., Ph.D., professor emeritus of medicine and biochemistry at the University of Nebraska College of Medicine in Omaha. "This biochemical oxidation process is not far removed from that which turns an old piece of metal into rust."

Wrinkled skin, shrinking muscles, weak bones and other signs of aging may, in large part, be caused by this destructive oxidation process, says Balz Frei, PhD, director of the Linus Pauling Insititute at Oregon State University.

Several vitamins fight free radicals. These include vitamins C, E and beta-carotene, a substance the body converts to vitamin A. "Taking these vitamins can be quite helpful as people get older," says best-selling author Jason Theodosakis, M.D.

Vital Vitamins

These are just some of the vitamins you'll want to consider taking, alone or in a multivitamin supplement:

Vitamin A: strengthens eyesight; fights respiratory infections; promotes healthy bones, skin, hair, teeth, gums. Natural sources: fish liver oil, liver, carrots, green and yellow vegetables, eggs, dairy products.

Vitamin B1: also known as thiamine. Promotes growth, aids digestion, nervous system, muscles, heart. Natural sources: yeast, whole wheat, oatmeal, peanuts, pork, most vegetables, milk.

Vitamin B2: also known as riboflavin. Aids growth, reproduction; promotes healthy skin, nails, hair; improves vision. Natural sources: milk, eggs, liver, yeast, cheese, leafy greens.

Vitamin B3: also known as niacin. Promotes digestion, healthy skin, circulation. Natural sources: liver, lean meats, whole-wheat products, avocados, dates, figs, prunes.

Vitamin B6: also known as pyroxidine. Aids absorption of proteins and fats; prevents nervous and skin disorders; alleviates nausea. Vitamin B6 has reduced menstrual pain in some studies. The vitamin apparently works by increasing production of neurotransmitters that inhibit pain sensations. B6 also has been shown to help with depression, irritability and other symptoms of PMS and menopause. Natural sources: brewer's yeast, wheat bran and germ, liver, cantaloupe, cabbage, milk, eggs, beef.

Vitamin B12: promotes red blood cells, energy, nervous system. Natural sources: liver, beef, pork, eggs, milk, cheese.

Vitamin C: antioxidant; protects against viral and bacterial infections, some cancers; heals wounds, burns, bleeding gums. "There is good evidence that supplements of ascorbic acid may be useful in combating both physical and emotional stress," says Hans Fisher M.D, chairman of the Nutrition Department at Rutgers University. Natural sources: citrus fruits, berries, green, leafy vegetables, tomatoes.

Vitamin D: aids absorption of calcium and phosphorous for strong bones and teeth; encourages assimilation of vitamin A. Natural sources: fish liver oils, fatty fish, milk, dairy products.

Vitamin E: antioxidant; protects lungs from air pollution; prevents and dissolves blood clots; accelerates healing from burns; diuretic. Vitamin E can boost immunity, reduce the risk of heart disease, cancer and cataracts, and alleviate Alzheimer's and Parkinson's diseases.

"We still don't know exactly how antioxidants such as vitamin E work to protect our cells from free radical damage," says Susan Mayne, Ph.D., associate director at Yale Comprehensive Cancer Center. "Vitamin E may mop up or neutralize free radicals and even repair some damage. Perhaps antioxidants transform free radicals into harmless substances or block steps in the disease process, such as in cancer."

In studies involving more than 100,000 health professionals, at least 100 IU a day of vitamin E were associated with a 40-percent lower risk of heart disease. And in a two-year study at Columbia University, researchers found that 340 people with Alzheimer's who took 2,000 IU of vitamin E daily delayed by seven months the loss of their ability to groom and feed themselves. Vitamin E may slow damage to brain cells.

Natural sources: what germ, soybeans vegetable oils, cruciferous vegetables, leafy greens, whole-grain cereals, eggs.

Vitamin K: powerful antioxidant effective for treating osteoporosis and other diseases. Natural sources: dark green vegetables, such as broccoli and spinach.

Magic Minerals

Minerals come in two categories. The major minerals—calcium, chloride, magnesium, phosphorous, potassium and sodium—are found in large quantities in the body and are abundant in food sources. Our bodies require large amounts of these minerals to keep us feeling young and healthy.

Trace minerals—chromium, copper, fluoride, iodine, iron, manganese, molybdenum, selenium and zinc—are found in much smaller amounts in our bodies and food. Our daily requirement for these minerals is lower.

Some minerals are stored in the body to replace those we lose in urine and sweat. But if we don't replenish minerals as rapidly as we deplete them, we run the risk of developing such diseases as iron deficiency anemia and osteoporosis.

The most important supplement for osteoporosis is calcium. Taking calcium can prevent and treat the disease, which causes your bones to become thin and brittle, and can lead to fractured hips and hunched spines.

And remember, you'll absorb more calcium if you take it with other nutrients. "Your body," for example, "can't absorb calcium unless you have plenty of vitamin D," says Michael F. Holick, M.D., Ph.D., of Boston University School of Medicine.

Among the minerals you'll want to consider taking, alone or in a multivitamin supplement:

Calcium: essential for strong bones and healthy teeth; keeps your heart beating. Unfortunately, up to 70 percent of ingested calcium is secreted. To retain calcium, take vitamin D and avoid animal products and excess sodium, sugar, coffee and tobacco.

Natural sources: dairy products, soybeans, sardines, salmon, dried beans.

Chromium: aids growth; may prevent diabetes; helps to prevent and lower high blood pressure. Natural sources: meat, shellfish, chicken, corn oil.

Copper: aids iron absorption for optimal energy. Natural sources: dried beans, peas, whole wheat, liver, shrimp and other seafoods.

Iodine: helps to burn off excess fat; promotes energy, healthy hair, nails, skin, teeth. Natural sources: kelp, onions, seafood.

Iron: prevents fatigue; promotes growth, disease resistance; prevents and cures anemia. Natural sources: liver, red meat, egg yolks, oysters, beans, oatmeal.

Magnesium: promotes healthy cardiovascular system, teeth, digestion, emotional equilibrium. Natural sources: figs, lemons, corn, almonds, dark green vegetables, apples.

Manganese: eliminates fatigue, improves memory; reduces irritability. Natural sources: nuts, green leafy vegetables, beans, egg yolks, whole-grain cereals.

Phosphorous: promotes energy, growth, healthy gums and teeth. Natural sources: fish, poultry, meat, whole grains, eggs, nuts, seeds.

Potassium: aids waste disposal, blood pressure. Natural sources: bananas, citrus fruits, tomatoes, green leafy vegetables.

Selenium: aids tissue elasticity, some menopausal symptoms; may protect against some cancers. Natural sources: wheat germ, whole grains, tuna, onions, tomatoes, broccoli.

Sodium: prevents sunstroke; helps nerves and muscles to function. Natural sources: salt, shellfish, carrots, kidney, bacon.

Sulfur: tones skin and hair; helps to fight bacterial infections. Natural sources: beef, dried beans, fish, eggs, cabbage.

Zinc: accelerates healing; prevents infertility, prostate problems; promotes growth and mental acuity. Natural sources: beef, lamb, pork, wheat germ, brewer's yeast, pumpkin seeds.

Understanding Hormones

If you've ever been around a teenager, you're familiar with hormones. Hormones are what makes kids act like they're crazy. They're vital for mood regulation, sex drive, sleep and a host of other functions.

Your body produces a number of hormones, but production slows as you age. Thus, you may not have enough for optimal health.

Hormonal supplements are commonly used to treat a number of conditions. Many women take replacement estrogen and other hormones during and after menopause. Travelers often use a hormone called melatonin to reset their "body clocks" and recover from the effects of jet lag. What's more, scientists are discovering new hormones all the time.

Researchers, for example, recently identified a hormone that reduces the desire to overeat. People who took it ate a third fewer calories than untreated counterparts. The hormone, PYY3-36, is released from the digestive tract after eating. It then travels to the brain and reduces the desire to eat again. The more calories you consume, the more hormone your body puts out.

"This is the natural way that the body turns off the appetite after a meal," says researcher Stephen R. Bloom at London's Imperial College of

Medicine. Bloom and colleagues injected study patients with the hormone and found that they could reduce their appetites.

Michael W. Schwartz, M.D., a researcher at the University of Washington, thinks that within five years we'll see a number of new medicines based on hormones and other natural supplements. "These drugs," he says, "should be much more effective than the ones that are now available."

All the Rest

Vitamins, minerals and hormones are fairly easy to understand. But what about the wealth of other supplements—many with arcane names—that line the shelves of health-food stores and pharmacies? If you decided to take all of them, you'd consume hundreds of pills a day—and spend the bulk of your pay check.

"Choosing the right supplements is vital," says pharmacist and author Mindell. But how do you know which are best for you?

Here's a look at the pros and cons of the top-selling supplements. Talk with your doctor about them. Then the two of you can decide which supplements, if any, you should take and in what dosages.

Arginine

The Up Side: Arginine, an amino acid, incites the pituitary gland to release growth hormone. It may strengthen the immune system, slow tumor growth, speed healing of wounds and burns, detoxify the liver and prevent loss of muscle after injury or surgery. Norwegian studies indicate that arginine increases sperm count.

The Down Side: High doses may cause diarrhea, nausea, skin thickening, and agitation. Because arginine releases growth hormone, don't give it to children.

Coenzyme Q10

The Up Side: Coenzyme Q10 (CoQ10) regulates electrical currents in the energy-producing mitochondria of our cells. Clinical trials from around the world strongly indicate that CoQ10 strengthens the heart, prevents and treats cancer (especially breast cancer), speeds recovery from illness or surgery, fights gum disease, and may help muscular dystrophy.

The Down Side: Extremely high amounts could cause upset stomach or diarrhea.

CoQ10 is so important to the future of disease prevention, that I am including a lengthy discussion of it here. Take a look at the diseases scientists have treated with CoenzymeQ10 and you'll understand why researcher Peter Lansjoen calls the organic substance "the most fundamental change in medicine since the discovery of the microbe."

Studies from around the world have contributed to the mounting evidence that CoQ10 may be effective in treating or preventing cancer, heart disease, muscular dystrophy, Parkinson's disease, chronic fatigue syndrome, periodontal disease and AIDS. CoQ10 can boost your energy levels and make you look and feel younger. In fact, it may even help you to live longer.

"It's not a panacea, but it is a substance that can do an awful lot of good for an awful lot of people," says researcher William V. Judy, a veteran CoQ10 researcher at the Southeastern Institute of Biomedical Research in Bradenton, Fla.

If that's so, then why aren't more doctors prescribing it? "The problem with CoQ10," Judy says, "is that it's a natural substance and, as such, not subject to patent laws. Therefore, the big drug companies haven't been interested in studying it."

In other words, pioneer researcher Karl Folkers said in an interview before his death in 1997, "The reason CoQ10 is not a household nutrient in the West has more to do with the lack of protected marketing positions than with its safety or how well it works."

What is CoQ10? Your body is composed of more than a trillion cells, each of which contains mitochondria. Think of mitochondria as energy-generating factories. Here nutrients obtained from the foods you eat are burned in the presence of the oxygen you breathe. In order to make energy, mitochrondria must have CoQ10 molecules, which assist several enzymes in stimulating the process.

Nobody had ever heard of CoQ10 until 1956, when scientists at the University of Wisconsin isolated a crystalline compound from beef heart mitochondria. They sent the sample to Folkers, who then was head of a biochemical research team at Merck Sharp and Dohme Research Laboratories in Rahway, N.J. It was Folkers who determined the chemical structure of the substance, which is found in high concentrations in the heart, liver, kidney and pancreas.

Scientists subsequently noted that CoQ10 levels were well below normal in patients who suffered from a wide variety of ailments, including heart disease, cancer and muscular dystrophy. One study of more than 1,000 heart attack patients, for example, found that their blood and tissue levels of the substance were markedly lower than those of healthy people.

Nonetheless, it was years before anybody conducted a major study of CoQ10. That's because no one could obtain enough of the stuff. Although CoQ10 is present in nearly all foods, as well as human and animal tissues, it was difficult and costly the extract.

Then in 1974 researchers at the Japanese company Nisshin found a way to produce CoQ10 from an ingredient found in tobacco. That discovery was followed in 1977 by development of fermentation methods to make the substance. The researchers called the coenzyme Ubidecarenone and began marketing it as a cardiovascular medicine. By 1982, Ubidecarenone had become one of the top-five-selling drugs in Japan, consumed daily by more than 6 million Japanese. That's not surprising when you consider the staggering range of ailments it may be effective in treating:

Heart Disease. Evidence is sound that CoQ10 strengthens the heart muscle. Not only can it protect you from developing heart disease, it can alleviate your symptoms if you develop cardiac problems, and possibly reduce your dependence on pharmaceuticals. A study in Germany found that CoQ10 is a powerful natural antioxidant, which can prevent cellular damage caused by heart disease. And more than 31 clinical trials in Japan alone have demonstrated the favorable effects of intravenous or oral CoQ10 therapy in patients who have suffered heart failure.

Cancer. Folkers and other researchers have discovered that CoQ10 may have significant use in combating tumors. The most compelling cancer study to date was conducted at a private clinic in Denmark and reported in 1994. Thirty-two patients with breast cancer were given a mixture of antioxidants (including vitamins C, E, betacarotene and selenium), fatty acids and 90 mg of CoQ10. After a month, six of the women showed signs of partial remission. Doctors increased the dosage to 390 mg. A month later, one woman's tumor had disappeared.

"I had never seen a spontaneous complete regression of a breast tumor with any conventional anti-tumor therapy," says Knud Lockwood, one of the principle researchers in the study.

Muscular Dystrophy. Double-blind studies have demonstrated CoQ10's effectiveness in treating muscular dystrophy. In one study, 12 patients ages 7 to 69 were treated for three months with 100 mg of CoQ10 and a placebo. The patients who took CoQ10 improved dramatically, while the placebo group continued to suffer progressive symptoms. As a result, researchers recommended, "Patients suffering from muscular dystrophies and the like should be treated with CoQ10 indefinitely."

Periodontal Disease. Doctors have observed that people with periodontal disease have significantly low levels of CoQ10 in the tissues of their gums. Researchers at Osaka University Faculty of Dentistry in Japan gave eight patients with moderately or severely inflamed gums 60 mg of CoQ10 a day for eight weeks. The patients received no other therapy. The results, according to clinicians: "CoQ10 was effective in suppressing gingival inflammation."

AIDS. People with Acquired Immune Deficiency Syndrome also have far less CoQ10 in their blood than healthy people. To determine the effect of CoQ10 in fighting the disease, Folkers and associates gave seven AIDS patients 200 mg of CoQ10 a day for several months. All seven started feeling better soon after beginning treatment. "The overall results," Folkers says, "were very encouraging and, at times, even striking."

Post-Operative Therapy. Post-surgical complications are a leading cause of death among hospital patients. That's because our bodies are vulnerable to any number of infections after suffering the immune system battering caused by a surgical procedure. But several studies indicate that people who take CoQ10 before they undergo operations recover much more quickly.

In an Italian study, for example, 40 patients about to undergo coronary artery bypass surgery were divided into two groups. Patients in the first group received 150 mg of CoQ10 a day for seven days before the operation; those in group two did not. Patients in group one recovered much faster than those in the second group, and suffered fewer complications.

"Our findings," the researchers said, "suggest that pretreatment with coenzyme Q10 may play a protective role during routine bypass grafting by attenuating the degrees of peroxidative damage."

Anti-Aging Formula. CoQ10 has three major functions: to help several mitochondrial enzymes convert dietary nutrients into energy; to quench free radicals generated in the energy-making process, and to help protect integrity of the mitochondrial membrane.

Because it is a powerful antioxidant—as powerful as vitamin E— CoQ10 may help you to feel and look younger, and live longer. Several studies have found that CoQ10 prevents oxidative stress in skin, protects sperm from oxidation and keeps them mobile, and slows the aging process.

Aging rats given CoQ10, for instance, developed the heart level function of young, healthy rats, according to Australian researcher Anthony Linnane. In another study, weekly injections of CoQ10 extended the life span of mice by 56 percent.

Until recently, scientists assumed that as we get older, out bodies make smaller amounts of CoQ10, which leaves us feeling weak and tired. But researcher Judy thinks something else may be going on.

"It may not be that our CoQ10 production goes down with age," he says. "It may be that we're using up all our CoQ10 to fight free radicals as an antioxidant, so there's not enough available to give us energy."

What's Ahead? Researchers say the evidence is overwhelming that CoQ10 is a vital nutrient necessary for health and well-being. English researcher Peter Mitchell, in fact, won a Nobel Prize in 1978 for his work in identifying CoQ10's attributes. But funding for clinical studies—from drug companies, the federal government and other sources—has been slow to materialize.

"Probably what will happen," Judy speculates, "is that 20 years from now somebody will rediscover this nutrient and patent a chemical analog. Then the pharmaceutical companies will become interested."

In the meantime, Judy says, researchers must wait. "And that's a real shame. There is so much more that we need to know about this substance."

DHEA (Dehydroepiandrosterone)

The Up Side: Levels of DHEA, a natural steroid hormone, decline as we age.

Boosting DHEA may improve immune function, memory, diabetes, low energy, lupus, depression and post-menopausal sex drive. DHEA also may protect against heart attacks and various cancers.

The Down Side: Until you reach age 40, your body does not need supplemental DHEA. After 40, take it only under a doctor's supervision. "Excessive levels of DHEA may stimulate the liver to produce male and female hormones that aren't needed," Adderly says. "An excess of male hormones could result in oily skin, mood swings, deeper voice, increased hairiness and even prostate cancer." Most hormone-related symptoms should disappear after you discontinue use.

Glucosamine

The Up Side: Glucosamine, a modified sugar molecule, encourages connective tissue to repair itself. "If you have osteoarthritis, you probably will experience excellent results by taking glucosamine," says Arnold Fox, M.D., an anti-aging expert in California. Glucosamine (often used with another supplement, called chondroitin sulfate) also helps to prevent breakdown of cartilage, says arthritis expert Jason Theodosakis, M.D. "There's quite a lot of evidence in Europe that these supplements are effective. Now the Arthritis Foundation in this country is seriously taking a look at them. And the National Institutes of health is doing a large-scale clinical trial on glucosamine and chondroitin."

The Down Side: Glucosamine appears to have no side effects.

Green tea extract

The Up Side: "Green tea is a rich source of polyphenols," says pharmacist and author Mindell. These compounds stimulant detoxifying enzymes that may block cancerous growth, and contain antioxidants more powerful than vitamins C and E. Unfermented green tea also contains potassium, magnesium and folic acid; catechins, which ward off viral infections and protect against various cancers; and fluoride, which prevents cavities. Consumed regularly, green tea also may lower risk of heart disease.

The Down Side: Green tea contains caffeine and other natural stimulants. Caffeine has been linked to insomnia, indigestion and fibrocystic breast disease.

Lycopene
The Up Side: Studies indicate that lycopene, a powerful antioxidant found in tomatoes and other foods, inhibits growth of cancer cells in the breast, lung and prostate. Cooked tomatoes contain more lycopene than fresh.

The Down Side: Lycopene is a relatively new carotenoid. No side effects are known.

Phenylalanine
The Up Side: Studies show that phenylalanine, which helps to manufacture mood-regulating brain chemicals, can lift depression, increase memory retention and heighten mental alertness. Phenylalanine also has analgesic and anti-inflammatory properties and may reduce pain and swelling.

The Down Side: Don't take this supplement if you have high blood pressure, skin cancer or the rare condition known as phenylketonuria. Also avoid the artificial sweetener aspartame, which contains phenylalanine. When mixed with antidepressant medications, phenylalanine may cause dangerously high blood pressure. Phenylalanine and tyrosine form tyramine, a substance that may induce migraine headaches. If you're susceptible to migraines, avoid the supplements, as well as tyramine-rich foods, including anything preserved, dried or fermented, such as jams, pickles, cheese, raisins and alcohol.

Phosphatidylserine (PS)
The Up Side: More than 60 published studies support PS's ability to boost memory by rejuvenating brain cells. PS, which functions like a telephone operator in conducting brain cell information, may turn back an aging brain's "clock" by up to 12 years. Four studies in the last decade indicate that PS may be useful for treating some symptoms associated with Alzheimer's disease.

The Down Side: A similar product called phosphorylated serine does not work like PS and could cause adverse reactions in some people. Read labels carefully.

Pregnenolone
The Up Side: Pregnenolone is produced by the brain and adrenal glands, but levels decline as we age. "Some studies suggest that by

restoring levels to youthful levels, memory and learning are enhanced," Mindell says. "Pregnenolone also has been used for arthritis."

The Down Side: Pregnenolone has no known side effects.

Dose: one 10-mg tablet daily

How to Choose a Supplement

Bewildered by the supplement boom? Here's some advice from the Council for Responsible Nutrition in Washington, D.C. Before trying supplements, assess your nutrition needs by asking yourself:

•How well do I eat?

•Do I select foods high in vitamins and minerals?

•Do I eat at least five servings of fruits and vegetables each day?

•Am I dieting or watching my calorie and fat intake?

•Do I smoke?

•Am I over 50?

•Am I taking medications on a regular basis?

•Am I pregnant or trying to become pregnant?

•Are there other health circumstances that may affect my nutrient needs?

•After you have compiled your nutrition profile, discuss it with your doctor. Then the two of you can determine whether you need to take supplements.

Supplement Sense

You've made the decision to take supplements. Now here's a plan of action:

•Start out by taking a balanced dose of vitamins and minerals—not just a lot of one or another. Take a broad-spectrum vitamin/mineral/ antioxidant supplement that provides up to 150 percent of the Recommended Dietary Allowances for nutrients. In addition:

•Choose a supplement with calcium. Women need at least 800 mg of calcium (and men need it, too, to prevent osteoporosis. The National Institutes of Health and the National Osteoporosis Foundation recommend up to 1,500 mg of calcium every day from foods and supplements.

For post-menopausal women, the average calcium intake from food sources is only between 560 and 600 mg a day, and many women fall below the 400-mg mark. In supplement form, calcium citrate appears to be the most absorbable form of calcium. And there is evidence that the citrate part of the molecule also may aid in preventing formation of calcium kidney stones.

•Choose a supplement with folic acid, if you're a woman. This is also called folate. This B vitamin has been shown prevent certain birth defects. But increased intake of folic acid now is recommended for all woman in child-bearing years. Taking folic acid can protect you from developing some forms of cancer, particularly cervical cancer. Take 400 mcg a day (up to 800 mcg if you're pregnant) and eat plenty of foods with folic acid, including leafy greens, beans, whole grains, broccoli, asparagus and citrus fruits.

•Avoid supplements with iron. Iron does help the blood to transport oxygen. But too much iron encourages formation of age-accelerating free radicals. Moreover, iron stays in your body. There's no way to get rid of it.

• Choose a supplement with antioxidants, especially betacarotene and vitamins C and E. These are extraordinarily safe, even if you take up to 10 times the daily RDA. Your supplement should contain six to 15

Supplements Action Plan

•**Viva vitamins!** If you do nothing else for your health, take a multivitamin once a day. How hard is that?

•**Supplement your diet.** Ask your doctor about disease-specific supplements. Most adults, for example, benefit from taking aspirin or garlic tablets, which ìthinî the blood and help to prevent heart attacks and strokes.

•**Consider CoQ10.** Studies from around the world indicate that this natural nutrient plays a significant role in preventing and treating everything from cancer to gum disease.

•**Try a supplement first.** Glucose levels tend to creep up as we grow older. If thatís a problem for you, consider taking chromium picolinate or vanadyl sulfate before trying a prescription medicine. The same goes for arthritis. Give glucosamine or chondroitin sulfate a try before risking side effects with prescription pills. Be sure to discuss a supplemental plan with your doctor before jumping in.

• **Peruse your prescriptions.** Are there any you take now that you might be able to replace with natural supplements? Ask your doctor for advice.

mg of betacarotene, 200-800 IU of vitamin E and 250-500 mg of vitamin C.

- Take low-dose aspirin. About 80 mg every day or every other day. It can reduce heart attack risk up to 40 percent; may reduce stroke risk 18 percent; may reduce colon cancer deaths by up to 50 percent; may reduce likelihood of migraine attack by 20 percent; may stave off certain forms of senility.

4. Exercise

Get Up and Go!

Regular exercise offers multiple benefits for body, mind and spirit. Just don't kill yourself trying to get in shape.

Actress Sharon Stone suffered a mild stroke while undergoing a grueling daily exercise regimen. Marathon runner Jim Fixx died while jogging.

For growing numbers of Americans exercise is almost an obsession. We've become a nation of gym junkies, punishing our bodies, pushing our willpower to the limit, in the relentless pursuit of the "perfect" physique.

But exercising excessively is *not* healthy. In fact, it can kill you or at least cause serious health problems. Researchers at Ohio State University, for example, have noted a 200 percent increase in exercise-related injuries and illnesses among people in their 40s.

Other studies, however, indicate that we're not exercising *enough*. New guidelines, in fact, suggest that if you want to get healthy and stay that way you need to exercise for at least an hour a day, double the previous workout recommendation.

"To reduce some of the main killers of America, we will have to increase the level of physical activity," says Dr. Benjamin Caballero, director of the Center for Human Nutrition at Johns Hopkins University in Baltimore.

It's frustrating when health experts contradict each other. No wonder, then, that some of us simply give up and plop ourselves down in front of the TV.

Let's Get Physical

As with any practice we undertake to achieve good health, exercise involves common sense. You don't need this book to tell you that it's good for you. Regular exercise, in fact, is essential for achieving and maintaining good health.

Numerous studies have concluded that regular exercise lowers blood pressure and increases metabolism. In addition, exercise tones your muscles and makes you look great. Exercise also can help you in your battle against pain from arthritis and other chronic conditions. That's because when you exercise you release endorphins, the body's natural feel-good chemicals. These block pain and keep you feeling happy.

But to get maximum benefits from physical activity, you have to exercise regularly. Riding a bike when you feel like it is fun, but you won't lose weight or strengthen your heart unless you ride regularly. Jogging and running as well get those endorphins flowing. But if you want to be healthy, you can't hit the track for a day or two and then give up.

Exercise every single day, even if it's just to walk around the block.

We have to exercise regularly to enjoy good health. But what does regularly mean? And who has time these days for anything extracurricular?

Caballero recommends an hour of moderate physical activity every day. Don't have an hour to spare? Not a problem. Caballero says that exercise time can be broken up and spread throughout the day. Certainly you can devote 15 minutes here and there to improving your health. And don't imagine that it won't make a difference.

"Every little bit of physical activity matters," says Michael F. Roizen, M.D., a gerontologist and professor at the University of Chicago and author of *RealAge: Are you as Young as You Can Be?*

What's more you don't need to hire a personal trainer, join a costly gym or health club or shell out hundreds of dollars for an exercise wardrobe. All you have to do is pick a physical activity you enjoy—and stick with it. Remember when you were a kid? Chances are nobody had to hold a gun to your head to get you outdoors. What did you enjoy doing then? Riding a bike? Hiking? Swimming? If you liked doing those things then, you're apt to enjoy them just as much now.

You'll never stick with an exercise program unless you enjoy the activity. Caballero recommends choosing fun activities, such as walking, slow swimming, leisurely bicycle riding or golfing without a cart.

Just don't overdo all that fun. Jogging, walking and running are great exercises to help you lose weight and tone your entire system. But how much fun is running until you're at the point of collapse?

Working out at the local gym also is a fine thing to do. Lifting weights, in fact, can keep you looking and feeling great in your 90s. But do you really have to be Mr. or Ms. Universe? How healthy is that anyway?

Too many of us, though, are pushing ourselves entirely too hard to have the perfect body, the perfect heart rate, the perfect blood-pressure reading. In reality, exercising too much will destroy your health, not improve it.

How do you know if you're exercising too much? It's probably pretty obvious to your family and friends. But if you need to be hit over the head, consider this: Symptoms of excessive exercise include loss of strength, speed, endurance and other elements of performance and appetite. Other symptoms include inability to sleep well, chronic aches and pains, soreness, injuries caused by overexertion, such as denidinitis, extreme fatigue, increase in resting heart rate and irritability.

"If you experience any of these you're probably doing too much and need to cut back and take a break," says exercise physiologist Richard Weil. Most people, he says, come back stronger than before if they take a five-to-seven-day break from strenuous exercise. "Of course, you can always remain active during the break," Weil says. "Just don't do vigorous exercise."

A brisk walk, in fact, may be all you need to maintain good health. A new study suggests that walking may be as good for women's hearts as a trip to the gym—providing that they do it regularly.

The study, published in *The New England Journal of Medicine*, found that postmenopausal women who walked at a moderate pace for at least two and a half hours a week reduced their risk of suffering a heart attack or stroke by nearly a third.

In addition, several studies conclude that regular exercise lengthens life span. In other words, the more you move, the longer you'll live—and those years will be filled with good health.

Moderate exercise is all you need to look and feel better.

> *Research shows that exercise adds youthful years to your life. "People who are physically active have the bodies of those who are eight years younger," says author and anti-aging expert Michael Roizen.*

Make Your Moves

There are two types of conventional exercise that will help you to feel and look better: aerobic workouts and resistance training.

Aerobic exercises boost your heart rate and put your major muscle groups to work. Popular aerobic activities include walking, hiking, running, jogging, dancing and biking.

The benefits of aerobic exercise are numerous. For one thing, it helps to decrease the risk of cardiovascular disease, the number-one killer of men and women in the United States, says Alan Mikesky, Ph.D, an exercise physiologist at Indiana University School of Physical Education in Indianapolis. Regular aerobic exercise reduces blood pressure and cholesterol and builds bone density.

"If ever there was a fountain of youth, this is it," says William Simpson, M.D., professor of family medicine at the Medical University of South Carolina in Charleston.

Resistance training, which involves lifting weights, also can help you to look and feel younger. And don't think you're too old to start lifting weights. Studies show that even the oldest subjects—people in their 80s and 90s—responded well to resistance training. Their muscles, in fact, grew in size and strength every bit as much and as quickly as they did in people young enough to be their grandchildren.

As with aerobic exercise, frequency is the key to resistance training. Do it every day and you'll improve muscle strength and endurance, qualities that enable you to enjoy the activities you love well into old age.

Weight training also can improve your cholesterol levels, enhance bone strength, help you to maintain or lose weight, and improve your body image and self-esteem.

"If people stay with it, continue to be active and continue to do activities that stress the muscles, they can fight off some of the effects of aging," says Mikesky. "People can continue to do the things they enjoy in life longer—and not only that, but also maintain their performance in what they're doing."

What's more, you'll see results quickly—in as little as two weeks. In a study at Indiana University-Purdue University, 62 older adults were put on a resistance-training program. In just a few weeks, they showed an average 82 percent increase in strength.

Can't bear the thought of sweating it out? There are other types of exercise you may want to consider. They're less strenuous and physically demanding, but they may be just the ticket for making you look and feel years younger.

Stay Young With Yoga

Yoga, a 4,000-year-old system of exercise and meditation from India, has 20 million followers in the United States—more than triple the 6 million enthusiasts in 1994, says Trisha Lamb Feuerstein, head of research for the Yoga Research and Education Center, part of the International Association of Yoga Therapists in Santa Rosa, California.

"In the 1960s yoga was an attempt to get a drugless high," Feuerstein says. "Now it's more about stress reduction. Also, a lot of the boomer population is hitting an age where jogging is hard on the body. People are looking for a form of exercise that is gentler."

Yoga strives to unite body and spirit. Exercise poses, called *asanas,* promote flexibility, relaxation, strength and inner peace.

But yoga isn't just about spiritual awareness. Numerous studies in India and the United States conclude that yoga offers many physical benefits. If you suffer from mild asthma or high blood pressure, yoga may reduce your need for medicine. It's also helpful for people who are suffering from diabetes, Parkinson's disease, cerebral palsy, Attention Deficit Hyperactivity Disorder and back pain.

"Yoga exercises stretch each joint in the body through a full range of motion,," says yoga instructor Suza Francina, who specializes in classes for people over 50 at her Ojai Yoga Center in California.

By limbering up, you feel younger, Francina says. "The accepted view of aging is that it's a process of stiffening, rigidity and closing down. Most Americans don't get proper exercise, so their bodies contract with age and they lose height, strength and flexibility."

Yoga also gives you a constant source of energy, says Alice Christensen, founder and executive director of the American Yoga Association in Sarasota, Florida. "When you practice yoga," she says, "you actually have more vitality and vigor. In that way, I really think it can help to make you feel younger."

Christensen's assessment of the ancient practice is corroborated by modern science. A study of 170 college students showed that those taking yoga classes had less tension, depression, anger, and fatigue after a class than before. And a British study finds that yoga breathing can reduce symptoms of asthma.

Yoga offers benefits to practitioners at many different levels, says Rolf Slovik, director of New York's Himalayan Institute of Buffalo. "People come for stress management or because they're trying to manage some physical problem. Some come because of a very strong spiritual curiosity. They want more quietness in their lives."

> *Yoga can help to improve your performance in other sports, such as golfing, distance running and even football, says Rebecca Laney, who runs the Center for Yoga and Health in Clinton, Miss. "It's an awareness of movement, weight distribution and posture. Developing such a sense can help athletes more clearly feel what they're doing."*

Meditation in Motion

Also from Asia is **tai chi**, a system of slow, deliberate movements from China. Tai chi can improve balance and help us to stay limber and stress-free as we age.

"Tai chi involves making very slow hand and arm movements," says Timothy Hain, M.D., associate professor of neurology and otolaryngology at Northwestern University Medical School in Chicago. "It's about controlling what you're doing."

Tai chi may prevent arthritis. "Because you move the whole body, including wrists, knees and other joints, tai chi keeps the joints lubricated. It is a smooth and relaxed form of exercise, very soft like a continuous dance." In addition, Hain has studied tai chi as a treatment for balance problems caused by inner ear disorders.

"Tai chi offers so many different ways to improve balance," he says. "There are movements that strengthen the legs. It's also a controlled way to explore your center of gravity."

Tai chi also boosts concentration, and it can reduce stress and lower blood pressure, says Tingsen Xu, PhD, a tai chi "grand master" who began practicing tai chi in his native China at age 15. Now in his 70s, he is an associate professor in the neurology department at Atlanta's Emory University Medical School.

"I call it meditation in motion. You erase everything form your mind, concentrate on movement. It is very much a mind-body connection. Fifteen to 20 minutes of tai chi every day can reduce that stress."

Move, Move, Move

It really doesn't matter which physical activities you choose. Just get up and move—even for only minutes a day in the beginning of your health program. Remember, it's a process. The secret of deriving health benefits from exercise to do it regularly—20 minutes a day, an hour every other day. It's up to you. Just do it.

Exercise Your Brain

Remember to exercise your brain as well as your body. Scientists are learning that if you have enjoy a vigorous lifestyle with a broad range of active intellectual interests, your mind will keep developing toward its full potential. That means you can be as sharp—or sharper—at age 70, 80 or even 90 as you were at 20.

In fact, a study published recently in the *Journal of the American Medical Association* suggests that regularly exercising your brain may help to protect against the devastating Alzheimer's disease.

"Best of all, it doesn't matter what age you are when you start," says Michael D. Chafetz, Ph.D., a research neuropsychologist at the University of New Orleans. "Improvement is always possible."

Here are some ways to give your brain a workout:

• Be more observant of people, places and objects that enter and leave your awareness each day. When you walk into a room, take note of the number and placement of people, furniture and other objects. Later draw a map of what you saw.

•Select a sentence at random from a newspaper, book or magazine. Then try to make another sentence, using the same words.

•Play games that challenge your reasoning skills, such as bridge, pinochle, chess, checkers, and crossword puzzles.

•Broaden your vocabulary by learning a new word every day.

•Ask, "What if?" and let your imagination soar.

•Be creative. Compose limericks or jokes.

•Lighten up. "Overwork is a prime cause of mental of impairment, " says Monique Le Poncin, Ph.D., a brain researcher at the French National Institute for Research on the Prevention of Cerebral Aging.

•Recite a poem while you jog.

•Weave your experiences into stories. Research indicates that human memory is story based. "Memory, in order to be effective, must contain both specific experiences and labels," says Roger C. Schank, Ph.D., director of the Institute for the Learning Sciences at Northwestern University in Evanston, Illinois. "The more information we are provided with about a situation, the more places it can reside in memory."

Exercise Your Spirit

Canadian researchers report that regular exercise may help many people who suffer from psychiatric disorders, including depression, which often strikes older people.

Researchers Gregg A. Tkachuk and Garry L. Martin. of the department of psychology at the University of Manitoba in Winnipeg, examined studies of anxiety disorder and exercise dating back to 1981. They found that strength training, running, walking and other forms of aerobic exercise help to alleviate mild to moderate depression, and also may help to treat other mental disorders, including anxiety and substance abuse.

"There is now considerable evidence that regular exercise is a viable, cost-effective but underused treatment for mild to moderate depression that compares favorably to individual psychotherapy, group psycho-therapy, and cognitive therapy," the researchers said in their study, which was published in *Professional Psychology: Research and Practice.*

Also, the researchers note, exercise may be an important component of treatment for body image problems, substance abuse problems, and somatic disorders in which mental symptoms manifest as physical pain.

Exactly how exercise helps to lessen depression and other psychiatric disorders is not fully understood. Improvements may result from a combination of factors, including release of endorphins. In addition, exercise may provide a distraction from negative emotions such as sadness and hopelessness, two hallmarks of depression. And exercise may help to buffer the effects of stress, which prevents illnesses.

Exercise Action Plan

•**Act up**. Make a list of activities you enjoyed as a kid: walking, running, biking, swimming. Pick one and give it a try as a grownup. Make it fun. Youíll never stick with an activity unless it brings you pleasure.

•**Try a new sport**. Ever wanted to play tennis or take up golf? How about one of those ìexoticî exercises, like yoga? Donít be afraid to try. Take a class. What have you got to lose—except your health problems?

•**Start off slowly**. Itís your life, not a marathon. Try 20 minutes a day and build from there.

•**Make a commitment**. Set aside a time when you will exercise each day. Then do it.

•**Boost your brain power.** Donít forget to exercise your mental faculties. Itíll keep you young. Solve a crossword puzzle. Learn a new language. Play a computer game.

5. Sleep

Snooze, Don't Lose

If you find yourself tossing and turning all night long, take charge and get a handle on your sleep habits. Getting a good night's sleep is essential to achieving good health.

If you're like most people you've spent at least one seemingly endless night, tossing and turning. Insomnia is one of the most common complaints in our stress-filled society. Getting a good night's sleep is essential to achieving and maintaining good health. But as we get older it gets harder and harder to sleep. Loss of sleep can make you look and feel years older than you really are.

The good news is that you can change all that. Even in your 90s you can enjoy a long, deep healthy night's sleep that will leave you feeling rejuvenated and ready to take on the world.

> *Sleep like a baby by eating wholesome foods, using healthy herbs and adding appropriate supplements to your diet.*

Why is a good night's sleep so important? "Sleep maximizes the quality of our lives," says Michael Vitiello, Ph.D., a sleep specialist at the University of Washington Medical School in Seattle. "When you sleep better you feel better, and all those things we associate with youth—appearance, energy and attitude—will ultimately improve."

Peter Hauri, Ph.D., a sleep expert at the Mayo Clinic in Rochester, Minnesota, says that sleep is interwoven with every facet of our lives. "It affects our health and well being, our moods and behavior, our energy and emotions, our marriages and jobs, our very sanity and happiness."

When we sleep we release the greatest concentration of growth hormone, the substance that helps to strengthen our bodies and repair damaged tissue. In addition, several studies show a close connection between sleep and the immune system. Sleep-deprived people, for example, experience a decrease in the activity of natural killer cells that keep the body healthy and infection-free.

Yet one of every three people develops sleep problems each year. And, because sleep patterns change as we age, sleep disorders frequently plague older people.

We spend nearly a third of our lives between the sheets. So why are as many as 40 million Americans afflicted with more than 70 types of sleep-related problems?

Doctors recognize three types of insomnia. People with sleep-onset insomnia have trouble falling asleep. Those with sleep-maintenance insomnia have trouble staying asleep, and if you suffer from early awakening insomnia, you may find that your eyes blink open long before the alarm clock shrills.

Many factors can contribute to insomnia: anxiety, inappropriate use of medications, physical conditions such as sleep apnea or restless leg syndrome, poor diet, and lack of exercise.

In addition, our society tends to be "high-strung," says James P. Kiley, Ph.D., director of the National Center on Sleep Disorders Research. "We have a society that's on a 24-hour cycle, with people having multiple jobs in many cases and multiple responsibilities both at work and home. When you're pushed for time, as many people are, the first thing that usually goes is sleep."

But when you sacrifice sleep, Kiley says, you're likely to end up paying for it—in decreased productivity and increased risk for errors in judgment and accidents. There's a strong link, for example, between lack of sleep and serious accidents.

Fatigue, as you know, leads to diminished mental alertness and concentration. Kiley estimates that there are as many as 1,500 fatalities and 100,000 sleep-related automobile accidents in the United States each year.

"The biological clocks of sleep-deprived people are ticking a the wrong times," he says. "They may drive home after work when they're extremely tired. Young males under 25 in particular have a number of auto accidents related to sleepiness."

So how do we get a good night's sleep? Not by taking drugs.

Dangerous Dreams

Prescription and over-the-counter sleeping pills will send you off to Dream Land. Each year, in fact, upwards of 6 million Americans obtain prescriptions for sedative hypnotics, many of which contain drugs called benzodiazepines, which work by reducing the brain's activity.

"For short-term use, these are very effective sleeping agents," says psychiatry professor Matthew A. Menza, M.D., of Robert Wood Johnson University Hospital in New Brunswick, New Jersey.

But prescription sleeping pills have serious drawbacks. They may cause increased tolerance, dependence, physical addiction, morning "hangovers" and withdrawal symptoms if you stop taking them. Another serious side effect is rebound insomnia. After you stop using some drugs, your sleep disorders actually may worsen. Benzodiazepines can make symptoms worse in some people who suffer from depression. Alcohol, moreover, intensifies the effects of the drugs; the combination, in fact, can kill you.

Over-the-counter sleeping pills, including antihistamines, also will help you to fall asleep—at first. But after a couple of weeks, most OTC remedies begin to lose their effectiveness.

Even more troubling is the warning from Konrad Kail, N.D., past president of the American Association of Naturopathic Physicians. Kail says over-the-counter and prescription sleeping pills appear to alter brain wave patterns of sleep, thus preventing you from getting a normal cycle of sleep stages, which is necessary for optimal health.

So what do you do if you suffer from a sleep disorder? First, discuss the problem with your doctor. Then consider some natural sleep strategies that may help you.

Sleep Strategies

Sleep disorder experts have plenty of tricks up their sleeves to help you get the 40 winks you need for a healthy lifestyle. Consider some of these:

Take it easy. Leave stress at the bedroom door. Breathing exercises may help. Exhale through your mouth, then inhale through your nose to a count of four. Hold your breath for a count of seven. Exhale through your mouth for a count of eight. Repeat the cycle three times.

Sleep central. The bedroom should be where you sleep, not where you read, snack, work or play. Make your bedroom a shrine to sleep. First, keep the room dark. Then get rid of the clock. "Set the alarm if you must," advises Hauri, "but put it where it can be heard but not seen." You might even try sleeping on linen sheets. Sounds kooky, but Italian researchers at the University of Milan report that people who sleep on linen fall asleep faster and wake up in better moods than those who slumber on cotton or other fabrics. Perhaps, the researchers theorize, linen sheets disperse body heat better than other fabrics. Finally, consider repainting your bedroom. Behavioral psychologists say that color influences our moods and may affect our sleep patters. Green, for example, seems to evoke feelings of serenity and lower the heart rate. Blue causes the brain to secrete tranquilizing hormones. Violet calms the nerves and slows muscular responses.

Turn up the heat. Sleep specialists at Northwestern University Medical School in Chicago have noted that many people can fall asleep if they use a heating blanket, which relaxes muscles and increases brain temperatures. It may help if you raise your temperature three to five hours before going to bed. "If you can increase your body temperature before going to bed, the temperature then will drop most as you are ready to go to sleep," says Hauri. Don't sleep under the blanket all night, though, or you may get too hot and wake up early. Instead, try a heating blanket with a timer that shuts off about an hour or two after you've fallen asleep.

Change your diet. Avoid coffee, tea and other caffeinated beverages within four to five hours of bedtime. But you knew that, didn't you? You also probably are aware that you should nix the nightcaps. Alcohol makes some people drowsy, but it also disrupts normal brain-wave sleep patterns and may prompt you to awaken frequently. Finally, don't go to bed hungry. If you eat an early supper and then skip a mid-evening snack, your blood sugar may drop in the middle of the night, prompting you to awaken.

Good evening snacks include low-fat cookies, air-popped popcorn, fresh fruit or sorbet, low-fat tea cakes and starchy foods, such as a plain-baked potato or a slice of bread. Milk moreover contains tryptophan, a natural chemical that induces sleep.

Move—but not too much. Get plenty of exercise throughout the day, but don't exercise strenuously after dinner. Concentrate on relaxation then.

It's all in the timing. Rise at approximately the same time very morning, and don't oversleep on weekends. That confuses your body's biological clock and lowers energy rather than raises it. "The worst thing in the world you can do is sleep in on a Sunday morning," says Charles Winget, Ph.D., a National Aeronautics and Space Administration scientist who is an authority on sleep cycles. "Essentially you're becoming jet-lagged. You might as well fly from California to New York." Go to bed around the same time every night. Avoid naps in the afternoon or limit them to less than an hour before mid-afternoon. If you can't fall asleep after 20 minutes, get up and do something else.

Here's a fun way to relax. Have sex. Sweet dreams!

Take a warm bath. It's not just an old wives' tale. Taking a warm bath an hour or two before you go to bed really will help you to sleep better. Like a fever, the bath spurs your brain's sleep-inducing mechanisms.

Positioning Yourself

How you place your body in bed may have a lot to do with the quality of the sleep you get. Experts offer this advice:

• Don't sleep on your stomach. It puts pressure on your abdomen and diaphragm, which can affect your breathing and cause a decrease in oxygen to your tissues.

• Don't sleep with your arms above your head. This pulls blood away from the heart and slows down return of blood to the heart. That makes the heart work harder and decreases oxygen supply to your heart and lungs.

• Don't sleep on your back. It can put stress on your back, which doesn't do much for your sleep. Sleeping on your back also is a problem if you have a hiatal hernia, asthma, gastro-esophogeal reflux, chronic sinusitis or postnasal drip. If you must sleep on your back, your head and upper back should be elevated slightly with a pillow.

What's the best sleep position:? One that doesn't stress spine, muscular system or nerves. In other words, the fetal position. Lie on either side, with legs flexed toward the abdomen and back slightly flexed.

This takes stress off the spine and allows organs to spread themselves out so there isn't so much abdominal pressure on the diaphragm. A pillow under the head or neck deflects weight from the shoulder you're lying on, so you don't run the risk of pinching nerves that run from your neck to your arms.

If you still have trouble falling asleep, talk with your doctor about trying an herb or supplement. Several have natural sedative properties to help asleep, with none of the dangerous side effects of prescription and OTC drugs.

Plant Pacifiers

Mother Nature knows that sleep is important for health. Many of the plants in her garden are great for lulling you off to sleep, and they work in a variety of ways. Certain scents produced by herbs, for example, seem to activate sleep-related chemical messengers, called neurotransmitters, in the brain. Try using these relaxing herbal oils ((5 drops in bath water or 2 drops on your pillow): chamomile, lavender, neroli, rose or marjoram.

Other herbs are best brewed as teas or taken in capsule form. **Valerian**, for example, has been used for centuries to help people fall asleep. Herbalist and author David Hoffman, in fact, calls valerian "one of the most useful relaxing herbs." Many Europeans would agree. More than 100 drugs based on valerian and its derivatives are marketed in Germany alone.

"Valerian enables you to relax both physically and mentally when you are overworked or experiencing tension and stress," says Peter Theiss, author of *The Family Herbal*, and founder of a large German pharmaceutical herb company. "It does so without making you tired, creating a narcotized sensation or causing dependency.

Alan R. Gaby, M.D., former president of the American Holistic Medical Association, recommends valerian for patients with mild to

Valerian on Trial

In study after study, valerian seems to work as well as benzodiazepenes in helping people to fall asleep.

•In one double-blind study, 44 percent of insomniacs who took valerian described the quality of their sleep as "perfect," and 99 percent said their sleep had improved significantly. None of the patients reported any side effects.

•In another experiment, 128 people with sleep problems were given either 400 mg of valerian root extract or a placebo. Those taking the herb reported significant improvement in sleep quality without morning grogginess.

•Valerian also significantly improves sleep latency, which is how researchers describe the time it takes a person to fall asleep. One study found that valerian halved the time it normally took volunteers to fall asleep.

•Another randomized double-blind study had patients with mild insomnia take either a placebo or an extract of valerian root. Subjective sleep ratings were assessed by a questionnaire and the patients' movements were recorded throughout the night.

The study found that valerian takers experienced a significant decrease in the amount of time it took them to fall asleep. Higher doses of valerian, interestingly, helped subjects to fall asleep no faster than moderate doses.

moderate symptoms of insomnia. "For those people, it's the first thing I try, usually in capsule form."

Valerian contains chemicals with strong muscle relaxant and sedative properties called valepotriates. All parts of the plant contain these chemicals, but they are most concentrated in the roots.

"Experimental results indicate that valerian root is at least as effective as small doses of barbiturates and benzodiazepines, without the side effects of the latter substances," says Daniel B. Mowrey, PH.D., author of *Herbs That Heal.*

Used in moderation, valerian has no side effects. What's more, valerian's sedative properties are not significantly exaggerated by alcohol, as are benzodiazepenes'.

Sleep Better With Supplements

Minerals, hormones and other supplements also may you to get the sleep you need to feel your best. For example, **calcium** (500 mg) or **magnesium** (250 mg) taken before bed may have a tranquilizing effect.

Also helpful for many people is **melatonin**, a hormone that regulates sleeping and waking patterns. We produce melatonin in the bean-size pineal gland nestled deep inside our brains, and also in the retinas of our eyes. Melatonin production is stimulated by darkness and shuts down in bright light (especially sunlight). Normally, the pineal gland starts increasing melatonin production around 9 p.m. Hormone levels peak between 2 a.m. and 4 a.m. and then return to normal daytime levels.

Infants produce a great deal of melatonin. But after we reach puberty, melatonin levels begin to decrease. As we grow older, the pineal gland calcifies. As a result, "You lose pineal cells. as much as 50 percent," says Dr. William Regelson, a professor of medicine at the Medical College of Virginia at Virginia Commonwealth University in Richmond, Virginia. "Associated with that loss is a fall in melatonin." Thus, taking melatonin supplements may help you to sleep as well as you did when you were younger.

Exactly how melatonin works is unclear. At a worldwide scientific gathering in Switzerland in 1997, Dr. Peretz Lavie reported that electroencephalograms taken during secretion of melatonin are similar to those induced by benzodiazepene drugs such as Klonopin.

But melatonin in no other way resembles benzodiazepines, according to a study that appeared two years earlier in the journal *Psychopharmacology.*

Several studies from around the world demonstrate that melatonin-replacement therapy may be beneficial for people who have trouble sleeping:

•In a 1995 study in Israel, older people with sleep problems were given melatonin two hours before bedtime for seven days. Then researchers monitored the subjects' sleep and wake patterns. Melatonin, the scientists concluded, was effective for improving sleep maintenance.

•A 1994 trial reported in the journal *Neuroreport* in 1994 found that melatonin helped insomniacs to fall asleep nearly two hours sooner than usual.

•A 1995 study in the *European Journal of Pharmacology* proved that melatonin even improves napping. Young adults were treated with 3 mg to 6 mg of melatonin or a placebo. Those taking melatonin reported that they were able to get to sleep sooner and stay asleep longer than placebo-taking subjects. The melatonin group members also assessed the quality of their sleep as "deeper" than normal.

•Another study, in the British journal *Lancet* suggests that controlled-release melatonin may help to stay asleep.

Melatonin doesn't just help you to sleep or recover from jet lag. Several researchers have concluded that the hormone is a highly effective antioxidant, more powerful than vitamins C and E. Antioxidants do battle against free-radical oxygen molecules, which scientists suspect are the culprits behind aging and its attendant diseases. Thus, regular melatonin use may help to slow down your body's biological clock and leave you looking and feeling younger.

Don't Be Sleepless in Seattle—or Anywhere Else

Sleep is one of your body's best defense mechanisms against disease. If you're sleep-deprived you run the risk of getting sick, not to mention

Time Travel

Melatonin not only helps you fall asleep, it's beneficial when you're traveling. Your body is equipped with a biological clock that regulates sleeping and waking. activities. Traveling across several time zones disrupts that rhythm, says Richard Dawood, M.D., author of *Travelers' Health: How To Stay Healthy All Over the World*. The result is jet lag, that feeling of exhaustion and disorientation you get when you wake up the next day in a strange hotel room.

What may help in those cases is taking melatonin the night before. Melatonin, a hormone produced by your body, is believed to help keep your biological clock ticking by regulating what's known as the circadian rhythm cycle.

injuring yourself while you're awake. It's essential that you get winks—and then some. But exactly how much sleep is necessary health?

Sleep experts at the National Institutes of Health recommend that most people get from seven to eight hours of sleep each night. This figure varies considerably, depending on your age and physical makeup. But if you're getting under six hours of sleep a night, you may be compromising your health.

Try the natural therapies in this chapter. Probably at least one of them will work for you. If you're still not getting quality sleep, discuss the problem with your doctor. He or she may refer you to a sleep specialist, who can help to treat your sleep disorder.

As the Greek philosopher Sophocles said, "Sleep is the only medicine that gives ease." So give yourself a little ease. You deserve a good night's sleep.

Sleep Action Plan

•**Throw out the sleeping pills.** Instead, try a calming herb, like valerian, or a natural supplement, such as melatonin.

•**Savor a soak.** Raise your body temperature by taking a warm bath and youíll find it easier to fall asleep.

•**Put a cork in it.** A drink may help you to fall asleep, but not for long. Alcohol disrupts natural sleep patterns. Instead of a nightcap, have a glass of milk, which contains sleep-promoting tryptophan.

•**Barricade your bedroom.** No stress allowed in here. Leave your worries at the door. In fact, say out loud before you enter the room: iThis is the place where I am relaxed.î You may feel silly a first, but itís an affirmation that could change your life.

•**Time yourself.** Get up and go to bed at the same times each day. Donít sleep in on weekends. Stick to the schedule. Your body will thank you.

6. Mind

How Do You Feel?

Mental and emotional health are every bit as important as physical health. Sometimes, in fact, it's better to begin a healthy lifestyle from the inside out.

Your heart is pounding. Your palms are perspiring. You can't catch your breath. In our fast-paced, sometimes frantic culture, we all experience anxiety from time to time. But anxiety is more than just an uncomfortable feeling.

Untreated, anxiety takes a terrific toll on our bodies. Several studies have uncovered undeniable links between stress and development of life-threatening illnesses, including diabetes, stroke, heart disease and cancer.

But alleviating anxiety is easier said than done. Benzodiazepines and other pharmaceutical stress relievers work effectively to reduce short-term anxiety. Taken regularly, however, such medications may cause serious side effects, including addiction—and even death.

Anxiety is the body's response to a distressing situation, which may be actual or imagined. Periodically, everyone experiences some degree of anxiety. But anxiety may be triggered by even vague notions of distress. When the alarm goes off repeatedly, you may be suffering from an anxiety disorder.

> *Mind matters. To improve your physical health you also have to improve your mental health.*

Those jittery feelings result after your adrenal glands release large amounts of adrenaline. At the same time the brain releases its own form of adrenaline, a chemical called norepinephine. This is a neurotransmitter that stimulates cells in the brain and other parts of the body. You may experience an increase in heart rate and your breathing may become shallow and rapid. In addition, your liver releases energy-stimulating sugars and your muscles may tense as you prepare for "fight or flight."

Problems may arise if our warning systems work too well. The anxiety alarm, in other words, goes off even if there's no significant threat: no panthers springing, no buffaloes stampeding. Instead, we're perceiving danger when work piles up on our desks, the car conks out or the kids are yelling their heads off.

Every time such stressors spur our alarms to kick in, our organs face damage from release of powerful chemicals. Unless we do something to temper our reactions to stress, we may eventually come down with stress-related illnesses, such as ulcers or high blood pressure, or we could develop crippling anxiety disorders.

Understanding Anxiety Disorders

In our high-voltage society, anxiety disorders are rampant, and they come in a staggering variety. Among the most common are:

Free-floating anxiety. Also known as generalized anxiety, this is a reaction to the stress we all face from living in an increasingly complex world. We may feel anxious for no apparent reason, or feel a sense of doom as we wait for the "ax to fall" or the "other shoe to drop." Generalized anxiety afflicts twice as many women as men, and is more common among adults than children. It also is difficult to treat because it has no identifiable source.

Obsessive-Compulsive Disorder. Obsessive-compulsives are compelled to act out irrational thoughts. They may, for example, feel an overwhelming need to repeatedly make sure that they turned off the coffee pot or locked the door at bedtime. In severe cases, obsessive-compulsives may spend hours indulging in repetitive behaviors, such as washing their hands or cleaning their homes.

Obsessive-compulsive disorder is characterized by obsessions that cause marked anxiety or distress and/or by compulsions that serve to neutralize anxiety. Obsessions are persistent ideas, thoughts, impulses or images that are experienced as intrusive and inappropriate and that cause emotional distress. Compulsions are repetitive behaviors or mental acts (praying, counting, repeating words silently). The goal of compulsions is to prevent or reduce anxiety or distress. The person feels driven to perform the compulsion to reduce the distress caused by the obsessive thought.

Usually at some point during the course of the disorder, the person recognizes that the obsessions or compulsions are excessive or unreasonable, but is powerless to change his behavior without intervention.

Panic Disorder. Panic attacks are characterized by a sudden onset of extreme fear or tension. If you've ever had a panic attack, you may have thought at first that you were having a heart attack. One of the symptoms of a panic attack is rapid heart beat and shallow breathing. Remember the "fight or flight" response our ancestors exhibited in the presence of danger? The same thing happens during a panic attack. Chemicals are released and symptoms of profound anxiety overtake your body.

No one really knows why panic attacks occur. They seem to run in families, so there may be a genetic component. Studies of identical twins, for example, show that if one twin suffers from anxiety, the other is likely to be anxious as well.

Panic attacks also may result from long-term suppression of anxiety, as some psychiatrists theorize. Perhaps you grew up in a dysfunctional family. You may have pushed down the anxiety you felt at the time. Then, years later, the anxiety erupts when you're least expecting it.

Phobias. Do you break out in a cold sweat when you take your seat on a plane, even though statistics conclude that flying is one of the safest forms of travel? Do you shudder when you see a snake, even though the likelihood of your being bitten by one is small to none?

Phobias are irrational fears that produce physical responses. Surveys show that phobias are among the most common psychiatric disorders. More than half of psychiatric patients, in fact, admit to suffering from at least one phobia. Fears of heights and animals were the most commonly represented simple phobias experienced by patients in a study at Massachusetts Mental Health Center in Boston.

People with severe phobias often go out of their way to avoid contact with the thing that frightens them. Agoraphobics, for example, may be afraid to leave their homes.

Post-Traumatic Stress Disorder. Sometimes repressed anxiety takes the form of post-traumatic stress disorder. This condition made headlines in the years following the Vietnam War, after battle-scarred veterans began to demonstrate bizarre, disturbing, or violent behavior during "flashbacks" to the horrors they experienced in the trenches and jungles of Southeast Asia. Thirty years ago, post-traumatic stress disorder was misunderstood by most people. Today we know that anyone who has undergone a horrific event—a catastrophic accident, child abuse, or rape, for example—may later develop anxiety-related problems with serious consequences.

You may never experience any of these anxiety disorders, but chances are you have been depressed at one time or another, or that you know someone who has. Depression is one of the most common mental illnesses in the world.

> *Depression is nothing to scoff at; it's a serious, often devastating disease. Depression is not a character weakness; it's caused by a biochemical imbalance. If you experience symptoms of depression for several weeks, seek professional help.*

How We Feel

Doctors describe depression as a mood disorder whose symptoms last at least two weeks, producing exaggerated, inappropriate feelings of sadness, worthlessness, emptiness and dejection.

To feel upset because of a job layoff, divorce, bankruptcy or loss of a loved one is a perfectly normal response. But sometimes depression strikes for no apparent reason. Then there may be a biochemical imbalance. In any case, overwhelming feelings of sadness can be crippling.

Consider some of the data on depression:

•Depression is prevalent in our culture. More than 10 million Americans are treated for depression each year. It strikes all ages and races, both sexes and all socioeconomic groups.
•Depression affects more women—1 in 5—than men: 1 in 15.

Are You Depressed?

Life events can get you down. If you're still down after two weeks, you may be suffering from clinical depression. You may experience one or several symptoms, gradually or suddenly. These include:

•Persistent feelings of sadness, irritability, hopelessness, pessimism, helplessness, worthlessness, guilt, emptiness.
•Unexplained crying, changes in sleeping and eating patterns, headaches, stomach upset or other physical problems, including weight gain or loss..
•Loss of self-esteem, interest in pleasure activities, sex..
•Difficulty concentrating, remember, making choices or remembering.
•Suicidal thoughts.

- If you ever have suffered from major depression, you have a 50-percent chance of developing symptoms again.
- Millions of depression cases are not diagnosed or treated. Doctors may treat symptoms of depression, including poor appetite, insomnia, and headaches, but overlook the underlying problem.
- Depression costs our society an estimated $44 billion a year, including $24.2 billion for lowered productivity and absenteeism at work and $12.3 billion for medical and psychiatric care.
- More than 18,000 people commit suicide each year; often depression is involved.

Scientists are just beginning to understand how the human brain works, but it's clear that depression and other anxiety and mood disorders are linked to neurotransmitters, chemical "messengers" that help to regulate our feelings. Chief among these is **serotonin**.

Serotonin is a chemical in your brain that carries signals from cell to cell. If your brain doesn't produce enough serotonin, those signals can't move at the proper speed or intensity. Serotonin also acts as a kind of master chemical that controls the activities of many important brain compounds, including those that govern muscle movements, alertness, mental activity and the ability to fall asleep.

Most of us start out with enough serotonin to function properly. But poor diet, lack of exercise, use of harmful substances such as caffeine or alcohol, and physical and emotional stress can rob your brain of serotonin, producing a range of serious complications.

Why do brain levels of mood regulators fall in some people but not in others? Genetics may play a role. Depression and other mental illnesses tend to run in families. Depression, for example, is more likely to be shared by identical twins: If one is depressed, there's a better than 50 percent chance that the other will be, too.

Environmental and psychological factors also may play a role. Some clinicians believe that attitude—feelings of pessimism or low self esteem—may determine whether we become depressed. Others think that some people simply have larger reserves of "happy" neurotransmitters in their brains, while others have not enough.

Of course, we all must deal with unpleasant events. Such incidents may cause brain levels of norepinephrine and dopamine to fall temporarily. People with naturally large reserves usually get through the troubling times with minimal difficulties, but those with low chemical may be more likely to fall into a depression.

> *If you're suffering from anxiety or depression, talking with a professional may help.*

Dealing With Disorders

Don't ignore the symptoms. Mental illness is a serious matter. If you're grappling with anxiety, depression or other emotional disorders you can't begin to live a fully healthy life style. If you think you're suffering from depression or another mental disorder, seek professional help. There are a number of things that may help you to feel like yourself again.

Psychotherapy

People with anxiety or depression may find it helpful to talk with a psychologist, psychiatrist or counselor about their symptoms, feelings, behaviors and concerns. This treatment approach may be simple, consisting of support and advice, or elaborate, involving extensive psychoanalysis. Options include one-on-one cognitive therapy and group therapy.

Often psychotherapy is effective in helping patients who have not responded well to drug therapy. Researchers in The Netherlands, for example, found that cognitive therapy worked well for subjects plagued by paruresis, a fear of urinating in the proximity of others. After receiving cognitive therapy for 18 weeks, the patients reported a significant reduction of symptoms. Moreover, the researchers found that the patients maintained their psychiatric gains after six months.

Group therapy also may be effective in treating phobias. In Lyon, France, 55 patients with social phobias received cognitive and group therapy. The patients were evaluated after six and 12 months. Researchers found that the patients showed statistically significant improvement.

If you're feeling somewhat depressed, talking about it may help. But so-called "talk" therapies may not do much for you if you're suffering from a major depression resulting from a biochemical imbalance in your brain. In that case, you may want to consider pharmaceutical medicines.

Conventional Drugs

Since serotonin was discovered 50 years ago, scientists have developed a number of potent drugs that prompt the body to produce the neurotransmitter. Today physicians and psychiatrists have many drugs at their disposal to treat depression, anxiety and other mood disorders.

Tricyclic antidepressants include Tofranil (imipramine) and Elavil (amitriptyline). Called tricyclics because of their three-ringed chemical structure, they work by altering the way the brain responds to norepinephrine and serotonin.

Monoamine oxidase inhibitors such as Nardil (phenelzine) and Parnate (tranylcypromine), act as "shields" to norepinephrine and dopamine, preventing their breakdown by enzymes.

Selective serotonin reuptake inhibitors, include Zoloft (sertraline), Paxil (paroxetine), and Prozac (fluoxetine), one of the most widely prescribed drugs in the world. SSRIs enhance or increase serotonin levels by preventing the hormone from being reabsorbed and "taken out of circulation."

These powerful medications have helped many people to regain their sense of emotional equilibrium, but they have potentially serious side effects and must be used with caution. Benzodiazepines, such as Xanax, for example, are highly effective tools for alleviating anxiety. But if you take benzodiazepines too long you may become addicted to them or suffer adverse reactions.

What's more, pills are not the panaceas we may have thought they were. Studies have shown that drugs are of no value in treating about 33 percent of depression cases. In another 33 percent of cases, the drugs were only a little more effective than placebos.

Drug Dangers

Pharmaceutical medicines have helped thousands of patients to recover their lives after suffering from depression and other mood disorders. But most such medicines also have severe side effects:

Alprazalam (Xanax): may cause abdominal discomfort, agitation, allergies, anxiety; may interact with other drugs, including antihistamines and antidepressants; may produce withdrawal symptoms if you stop taking it abruptly.

Clonazepam (Klonopin): may cause behavioral problems, drowsiness, lack of muscle coordination; may interact with other drugs; may cause withdrawal symptoms.

Diazepam (Valium): may cause drowsiness, fatigue, lightheadedness, loss of muscle coordination; may interact adversely with other drugs, including antidepressants; may be habit forming.

Fluoxetine (Prozac): may cause diarrhea, nervousness, sleepiness, inability to sleep, headaches, chills, fever, chest pain, nightmares, decreased sexual drive, menstrual difficulties, tremors, nausea, vomiting, increased appetite, rapid heart action, abdominal pain, and difficulty in breathing.

Imipramine (Tofranil): may elevate or lower blood pressure and cause strokes, irregular heartbeat, anxiety, delusions, insomnia, seizures, nausea, vomiting, abdominal cramps, impotence, and altered liver function.

Lorazepam (Ativan): may cause dizziness, sedation, unsteadiness, weakness; if you suddenly stop taking it you may experience withdrawal symptoms.

Paroxetine (Paxil): may cause problems with erections and ejaculation, as well as weakness, sleepiness, dry mouth, dizziness, inability to sleep, sweating, anxiety, decreased appetite, and nervousness.

Setraline (Zoloft): may cause weight loss, insomnia, heart palpitations, dizziness, chest pain, mania, dry mouth, headaches, and sweating. Tofranil may elevate or lower blood pressure, and cause strokes, irregular heartbeat, anxiety, delusions, insomnia, seizures, nausea, vomiting, abdominal cramps, impotence, and altered liver function.

Tranylcypromine (Parnate): may cause anxiety, weakness, dizziness, nausea, abdominal pain, anorexia, chills, blurred vision, and impotence.

> *Don't want to take pills? Talk with your doctor about trying some of the many natural therapies that may alleviate symptoms of anxiety, depression and other disorders.*

Meditate and Move

Ironically, you may improve your mood by employing two seemingly contradictory methods: slowing down and moving faster.

Meditation and **deep-breathing** techniques help you to slow down. People who learn to perform these exercises teach themselves to quiet and clear the mind of "clutter."

Several clinical studies have shown that during meditation the body is altered in ways that are beneficial for people who suffer from anxiety. For example, the rate of metabolism drops and blood pressure decreases. Meditation may be performed daily, several times a week or just before a situation that might provoke anxiety.

Physician Andrew Weil, M.D., does deep-breathing exercises twice a day. "I do it in the morning, before I meditate, and in the evening, when I am lying in bed, just before going to sleep," says Weil, author of *8 Weeks to Optimum Health*. "I think of it as a kind of tonic, with wonderful effects on the involuntary nervous system."

Breathing deeply and meditating appear to decrease anxiety and help the body's systems to function better. The practices also may help to ease symptoms of several illnesses and uncomfortable conditions, including high blood pressure, cold hands, irritable bowel syndrome, benign cardiac arrhythmias, anxiety and panic disorders.

"It is the most effective and time-efficient relaxation method I know," Weil says.

Take a Deep Breath

Andrew Weil, M.D. recommends this breathing technique, adapted from ancient yogic traditions.

Sit quietly, with your back straight. Touch the tip of your tongue to the upper front teeth, then slide it just above your teeth, between the teeth and the root of the mouth.

Exhale through your mouth, making a "whoosh" sound. Close your mouth and inhale quietly through your nose to a silent count of four. Hold your breath for a count of seven. Exhale audibly through your mouth to a count of eight.

Repeat four cycles, then resume breathing normally. Do this at least twice a day.

It's also important for mental and emotional health to keep active. Canadian scientists report that regular exercise may help many people who suffer from psychiatric disorders.

Psychology researchers Gregg A. Tkachuk and Garry L. Martin at the University of Manitoba in Winnipeg, examined studies of anxiety disorder and exercise dating back to 1981. They found that strength training, running, walking and other forms of aerobic exercise helped to alleviate mild to moderate depression, and also may help to treat other mental disorders, including anxiety and substance abuse.

"There is now considerable evidence that regular exercise is a viable, cost-effective but underused treatment for mild to moderate depression that compares favorably to individual psychotherapy, group psychotherapy, and cognitive therapy," the researchers said in their study, which was published in *Professional Psychology: Research and Practice.*

In one study cited by the researchers, people who ran, walked or performed strengthening exercises three times a week for 20 to 60 minutes were significantly less depressed after five weeks. What's more, their gains lasted for up to a year.

The Canadian researchers also reported that exercise is more effective than placebos at reducing symptoms of panic. In one study of 46 people with moderate to severe panic disorder, those who ran three times a week for 10 weeks and those who took anti-anxiety medications felt better than people who took placebo medicines.

Studies included in the Canadian review also showed that exercise may help to treat symptoms of schizophrenia, a psychiatric disorder marked by delusions, confusion and emotional turmoil. However more studies are needed to confirm these findings, the researchers noted.

In the meantime, the researchers said, exercise may be an important component of treatment for body image problems, substance abuse problems, and somatic disorders in which mental symptoms manifest as physical pain. And exercise, they said, is an effective short-term treatment for reduction of destructive behavior and for increasing work performance in people with developmental disabilities, such as attention deficit disorder, which is marked by an inability to concentrate and hyperactivity.

Exactly how exercise helps to lessen depression and other psychiatric disorders is not fully understood. Improvements may result from a combination of factors, including release of brain chemicals called endorphins. Endorphins produce calming, soothing effects. In addition, exercise may provide a distraction from negative emotions such as sadness and hopelessness, two hallmarks of depression. In addition, exercise may help to buffer the effects of stress.

Eat and Be Merry

Simply making some healthful improvements to your diet may enable you to deal better with emotional and mental problems. Brain cells are hungry cells, demanding nourishment from as much as 30 percent of circulating blood. If the brain doesn't get nutrients, its biochemistry changes, resulting in fatigue, depression, irritability and other symptoms.

If you are feeling anxious or depressed, consider following these dietary guidelines:

•**Avoid alcohol**. It may seem to perk you up at first, but alcohol is a depressant, the last thing depressed people need. If you must drink, limit yourself to one drink per day— one and a half ounces of liquor, four ounces of wine or 12 ounces of beer.
•**Quit caffeine**. You may think it gives you energy, but caffeine can drain you mentally and physically. Give it up or cut back significantly.
•**Shun sugar**. Sugar jolts us with a sudden burst of energy, but when the body responds by snatching the excess sugar out of circulation, it often takes too much, leaving us feeling tired and depressed.
•**Consider the benefits of fish oil**. Researchers have found that the fatty oil in salmon, cod and other types of fish may alleviate symptoms of manic depression. The chemicals in the fish oil that seemed to help patients were omega-3 fatty acids, found in many types of fatty fish, as well as in canola and flaxseed oils. Scientists think that omega-3 fatty acids boost levels of serotonin in the brain, just like Prozac.

Vitamins and Minerals

Just as they help the body to heal physical wounds, vitamins and minerals can aid in recovery from mental and emotional ailments. Here are some you may want to consider:

Vitamin B1. This may help to alleviate side effects caused by antidepressant drugs, including dry mouth, insomnia, and stomach upset. Food sources include kale, spinach, turnip greens, green peas, lettuce and cabbage.

Vitamin B2 (riboflavin). In 1973 researchers discovered that healthy men developed symptoms of depression if their diets were devoid of this vitamin. Food sources include asparagus, broccoli, spinach and whole wheat bread.

Vitamin B3 (niacin or niacinamide). The body needs this vitamin to convert the amino acid tryptophan into serotonin. As far back as the 1950s, doctors were treating schizophrenics with B3. Many showed considerable improvement. If you take supplements and notice a red "flushing" on the skin of your face or neck, gradually decrease the dosage, per your doctor's instructions. You'll also find "non-flush" supplements at the health-food store or pharmacy.

Vitamin B5 (pantothenate). This helps the body to convert dietary choline into the neurotransmitter acetylcholine. Getting more choline to the brain may alleviate symptoms of depression.

Vitamin B6 (pyridoxine). You also need this vitamin to convert tryptophan to serotonin. You'll find it in brewer's yeast, sunflower seeds, soybeans, walnuts, lentils, lima beans, hazelnuts, brown rice and avocados.

Vitamin B12 (cobalamin). Your body needs only small quantities of this vitamin, but deficiencies may cause depression and confusion. B12 appears to fight depression by inhibiting monoamine oxidase (MAO), an enzyme that attacks certain neurotransmitters that help to elevate mood. In that sense, B12 works like the MAOI (monoamine oxidase inhibitors) drugs prescribed for depression. You'll find good amounts of this vitamin in beef liver, chicken liver, clams, oysters and sardines, with smaller amounts in eggs, many fish and cheeses.

Choline. A member of the B-family of vitamins, choline is converted by the body to acetylcholine, which plays an important role in learning and memory. Choline is more effective when taken with vitamin B5, which helps to "push" it into the brain. Choline-containing foods include eggs, brewer's yeast, soybeans, peanuts, green peas and peanuts.

Folic acid. Another B-family vitamin, folic acid has been linked to depression in a number of studies. Folic acid deficiency , in fact, is common in a number of psychiatric disorders. Many studies have examined folic acid's ability to fight depression. Food sources include bananas, green leafy vegetables, such as spinach, whole wheat bread and wheat germ.

Vitamin C. A deficiency of this vitamin quickly leads to depression and confusion. When researchers compared the amount of vitamin C in the blood of 885 psychiatric patients and 110 healthy controls, the psychiatric patients were found to have significantly less of the vitamin in their blood. Good dietary sources include chili peppers, guavas, parsley, green and sweet red peppers, broccoli, strawberries, oranges, mangoes and cantaloupes.

Potassium. Many symptoms of depression have been associated with low levels of this mineral. Low levels of potassium in the brain have been found in suicide victims. Replenishing potassium stores helps to reverse the fatigue and muscle weakness that may be associated with depression. Food sources include bananas, nonfat milk, oranges and peas.

Many herbs have been used for centuries to treat depression and other mood disorders. Talk with your doctor about trying some.

Feel Better With Herbs

As I've shown in Chapter 2, herbs are good for preventing and treating illness and promoting general well-being; in this section you'll discover how several herbs act directly on the nervous system, promoting relaxation and feelings of tranquillity. Other herbs may relax tense muscles, ease stress-related headaches, soothe stomachs upset by stress, and encourage restful sleep. These may be taken as a tea made from fresh or dried herbs, as an extract or tincture, or in capsule form.

St. John's Wort. Europeans have used this herb for decades to treat depression. In Germany, where its use is covered by health insurance as a prescription drug, some 20 million people take it. The main component in St. John's wort is a chemical called hypericum. It takes a while for the effects of hypericum to be felt. Many patients notice a change in two to three weeks, but others take up to six weeks to feel better.

The herb's side effects are mild and may include slight gastrointestinal irritation and fatigue. You may have heard about the sheep in Australia that grazed on St. John's wort and came down with serious sunburns. It's true that large amounts of hypericum may cause some sun sensitivity in light-skinned people. Taken under the supervision of your doctor, though, you're unlikely to experience dangerous side effects such as this.

St. John's wort appears to be quite effective in treating depression naturally. A review of 23 clinical trials involving 1,757 people with mild or moderate depressive disorders showed that St. John's wort worked as well as standard antidepressant drugs. Side effects occurred in only 19.8 percent of patients taking St. John's wort, compared with 52.8 percent of those taking conventional drugs.

Ginseng. This ancient remedy long as been prized in the Orient as a tonic and rejuvenator. Some scientists consider the ginseng root to be an adaptogen, a substance that helps the body to adapt to stress.

Ginkgo. The leaves of this tree increase blood flow to the brain. Several studies suggest that ginkgo may help people suffering from cognitive problems, Alzheimer's disease and depression.

Kava kava. Native to the islands of the South Pacific, this member of the pepper family induces feelings of calmness and serenity. "If my patients are on Xanax or Valium, I'll try to switch them to kava kava without exception," says Arnold Fox, M.D., a California-based cardiologist. "Taken as directed, kava kava is safe and often produces quite satisfactory results."

Just how kava kava works is unclear. Scientists have isolated several compounds from kava kava root. Called kava pyrones, these include kawain, dihydrokawain, methysticin, dihydromethysticin, yangonin, and dihydroyangonon.

Several laboratory trials have demonstrated that kava kava has a marked ability to calm jangled nerves. German researchers also have found that kava kava induces deep muscle relaxation, modulates emotions and promotes sleep as effectively as synthetic tranquilizers.

Overconsumption of the herb has caused a condition known in the Polynesian islands as "kawaism." Regular and prolonged use of kava kava may result in a yellow skin rash, which goes away after you stop using the herb. But kava kava appears to be quite safe when used in moderation.

"If stress is a problem in your life, kava kava really can make a difference," Fox says. "What's more, I think we're going to hear a lot more about kava kava in coming years. It's a remarkable herb with a great deal of potential."

Skullcap. Used extensively by Native Americans, this herb reduces anxiety and promotes sleep.

Valerian. The root has a calming, sleep-inducing effect on most people.

Supplements for Serenity

Several natural supplements also show promise for treating symptoms of depression and other emotional disorders. See Chapter 3 for more details about supplements in general.

DHEA. Also known as dehydroepiandrosterone, this hormone is produced in the ovaries, and in the glands of women and men. It's important for good brain function; the brain contains six and a half times more DHEA than any other organ. From puberty, DHEA levels rise steadily, peaking at about the age of 25. By age 70 or 80, there is only about 10 percent of that peak amount left. In several studies, DHEA has been shown to relieve depression, enhance memory and help people to deal with stress. Side benefits include strengthening the immune system, reducing body fat, lower blood pressure and reducing the insulin needed by diabetics.

DLPA. This supplement combines two forms of phenylalanine: d-phenylalanine and l-phenylalanine. The mixture works well to combat depression. In a landmark study in 1978 researchers gave DLPA to more than 400 patients suffering from various types of depression. Two weeks later, all depressive symptoms had vanished in 73 percent of those suffering from major depression.

DMAE (dimethylaminoethanol). This is a nutrient found in sardines and other foods. DMAE passes through the blood-brain barrier to the brain, where it helps to increase levels of acetylcholine, one of the neurotransmitters that affect mood and energy levels. DMAE been shown to elevate mood and improve memory and learning, It's even more effective when taken with vitamin B5 (pantothenate). DMAE has also been used with great success in the treatment of ADD (attention deficit disorder) in children and adults.

5-HTP. Europeans use this supplement, also known as 5-hydroxytryptophan, to treat depression, sleep disorders, obesity and other problems. "In my practice as a licensed physician, I have prescribed 5-HTP as part of an overall therapy program for hundreds of patients," says Michael Murray, N.D., author of *5-HTP: The Natural Way to Overcome Depression, Obesity, and Insomnia*. "The results have been tremendous: improved mood, better physical vitality, higher energy levels, and a rediscovery of the basic joy of being alive."

5-HTP, a compound produced by the body from tryptophan, can boost serotonin levels safely in many people. From the food you eat, molecules are broken down into nutrients, including tryptophan. Tryptophan is converted to 5-HTP, a powerful antioxidant your body needs to produce serotonin.

Evidence is mounting that 5-HTP supplements may help many people to overcome a wide range of serotonin-related illnesses. Not only does 5-HTP raise serotonin levels, which can help with mood swings, it also boosts levels of endorphins, the body's natural pain fighters.

L-carnitine. This amino acid has alleviated depression in some people and improved cognitive abilities.

Pregnenolone. Another hormone produced by the ovaries and adrenal glands, pregnenolone may be useful in treating depression. Some studies have shown that depressed people have less-than-normal amounts of pregnenolone in their spinal fluid. Pregnenolone likely works by preventing the brain from being overwhelmed by GABA (gamma aminobutryic acid) and other hormones that slow its activity. Other studies have shown that giving this hormone to older men and women improves their memory and concentration.

SAMe (S-adenosylmethionine). This is a natural metabolite produced from the essential amino acid methionine and adenosine triphosphate (ATP) by an enzyme known as MAT (methionineadenosyltransferase). It's in every cell in the body and plays an important role in critical biochemical processes.

When compared with antidepressant drugs, SAMe works faster and more effectively, with virtually no adverse side effects. In fact, unlike FDA-approved antidepressants that have side effects, SAMe produces side benefits, such as improved cognitive function, protection of liver function, and a potential slowing of the aging process. The major drawback of SAMe is that it is a difficult-to-produce natural substance with high manufacturing and packaging costs.

Tyrosine. The body uses tyrosine to make the neurotransmitters dopamine, norepinephrine and epinephrine, which play a role in elevating mood and keeping us alert. You'll find it in fish, poultry and other foods.

Mind Action Plan

•**Go on a journaling journey.** Keep a stress diary. Take a look at whatís really bothering you. Is it your job—or a personal problem you've been ignoring?

•**Take up a hobby**. Get your mind off your troubles. Paint a picture, play an instrument, crochet an afghan, collect stamps.

•**Talk about it**. If you're stressed to the max, it helps to get it out. Talk with your doctor, your minister, your spouse, your best friend. Chat online. Consider seeing a therapist.

•**Hush up**. Turn off the internal chatter. Quiet your mind. Try meditation—just five minutes a day, if you can't manage more. You needn't join a monastery. Teach yourself. It's not brain surgery. There are plenty of books and tapes out there.

•**Cultivate natural harmony**. Ask your doctor about herbs and supplements that can help you to deal with stress. Consider St. John's wort for depression; kava kava to improve your moods; ginseng to help you deal with stress.

7. Spirit

Do Some Soul Searching

No matter what you call it – spirit, soul, higher self – there is an indescribable essence within that needs to be cherished and nourished if you are to enjoy overall good health.

Having a healthy spirit is every bit as important as having a healthy body. Researchers at Arizona State University have concluded that a strong sense of spirituality is among the best predictors of well-being. In addition, more than 250 studies at Yale, Duke Dartmouth and other universities suggest that spiritual people enjoy:

•A stronger immune system.
•Lower rates of hypertension, heart disease, emphysema and depression.
•Greater mental and physical ability to deal with illness and recover faster.

"Spiritual belief is a powerful force, and doctors cannot afford to ignore it," says Herbert Benson, M.D., a cardiologist at Harvard Medical School.

What is spirituality? It's your attitude about yourself, the people around you, the Universe, life. How can your attitude about life affect your health? During stressful situations, the adrenal glands flood the body with chemicals that raise heart rate and blood pressure. Praying, meditating and reading uplifting literature appear to lower those chemical levels and prevent stress from harming our bodies.

> *Healthy people look and feel years younger than they are. But you can't enjoy true health unless you're healthy in spirit, says psychologist and author Thomas Moore. "A spiritual life of some kind," he says, "is absolutely necessary for psychological health."*

In the new millennium growing numbers of Americans are searching for meaning in a world that frequently seems meaningless. Traditional values and extended families no longer form the glue that holds society together. What binds us today are TV screens and computer terminals. As a result, psychologists say, more of us are feeling that something essential is missing from our lives.

"The great malady of the 20th century is loss of soul," says psychologist Thomas Moore, author of the best-selling *Care of the Soul*. "When soul is neglected it doesn't just go away; it appears symptomatically in obsessions, addictions, violence and loss of meaning."

The question is, how do we become more spiritual? How do we infuse our lives with meaning, give back to others, make the world a better, safer, healthier place?

> *Developing a sense of spirituality isn't as difficult as it may seem. You don't have to go to church or even believe in a god. All you have to do is change the way you view the world and the circumstances in which you find yourself.*

12 Steps to Spiritual Health

Moore and other experts aren't suggesting that we give up our secular lives and join monasteries or convents. They're not even suggesting that we develop any religious beliefs at all—although if you have them and they work for you, by all means, expand on them.

Otherwise, refocusing your outlook just a bit can help you to feel more connected to the world. Consider taking a few of these simple steps to put you in touch with your higher self:

1. Clean up your act. The Dalai Lama does not spend his free time on the couch with a bag of potato chips. Nourish your body with whole grains and fresh fruits and vegetables. Get adequate rest. And if you walk just 15 minutes a day you'll notice a dramatic improvement in your outlook as well as your physical health.

2. Define what spirituality means to you. If you're so inclined, return to the church of your childhood to rediscover your religious roots, or visit other churches and develop new traditions. Talk with friends of other faiths and find out what inspires them. Broaden your perspective by reading from the *Bible, Koran, Tao Te Ching, Talmud* or *Bhagavad Gita.* If religion turns you off, try uplifting secular literature, including *The Little Prince* by Antoine de Saint-Exupery, *The Prophet* by Kahlil Gibran, *The Road Less Traveled* by M. Scott Peck, or the poetry of Emily Dickinson.

3. Keep a spiritual journal. "Writing can help you pay attention to life's daily events and become aware of patterns or spiritual longing and aspirations," says Timothy Jones, former minister and author of *The Art of Prayer.*

4. Turn off the TV. Trade sitcoms for soothing music, at least for an hour a day, play games with your family or simply enjoy a conversation with a friend.

5. Stretch and surrender. Take up a spiritually based exercise, such as yoga or *tai chi.* Enroll in a class or teach yourself with books and videos. Or just make time each week to walk in the woods or a park. "Being out in nature can have a tremendous uplifting impact on how we see our lives," says Elaine St. James, author of *Inner Simplicity.*

6. Be still. Try to spend 15 minutes a day just sitting quietly, thinking of nothing, or take small breaks throughout your day to relax and breathe deeply. One study found that after meditating, 75 percent of insomniacs could sleep; 36 percent of women with unexplained fertility problems became pregnant; and patients with chronic pain felt so much better that they decreased their doctor visits by more than a third.

7. Talk to the universe. Prayer can be a powerful healing force. Researchers at San Francisco General Hospital found that cardiac patients who were prayed for recovered faster — even though they were unaware of the intervention. In lieu of prayer, try affirmations. Each morning look in the mirror and tell yourself: "I am happy and full of health."

Remember to accentuate the positive. Pay attention to the way you talk to yourself. Do you tend to use "negative" words, such as "can't," and "shouldn't."? Just for one day strike those words and phrases from your vocabulary and express only positive thoughts. Chances are you'll feel healthier at the end of the day.

8. Give of yourself. Volunteering is a great way to share your spirituality with the world.

9. Develop rituals. Mindful acts help us to attune with spirit. Try lighting a candle and burning a stick of incense as you soak in a steaming tub.

10. Practice random acts of kindness. Do an anonymous favor for a coworker. Allow another driver to pull ahead of you in traffic. Hold the door for a stranger.

11. Rejoice. The best way to maintain your spirituality is to count your blessings. Keep a gratitude list of everything that's right about your life. You'll be surprised by how many things you come up with.

12. Leave the world behind. Bypass the beach, the theme parks, the cities teeming with traffic. Instead take a vacation that will help you to become more spiritual.

Spirited Getaways

Growing numbers of travelers are transforming their vacations into epiphanies. Instead of basking on a beach or trudging from one museum to another, they are seeking meaning by meditating on mountain tops, studying ancient shamanic rituals, making pilgrimages to holy sites, practicing yoga at holistic retreat centers and sitting in silence at Zen monasteries.

Spiritual travel attracts people from all walks. They may be undergoing major life changes: divorce, job loss, or mid-life crisis. But anyone can benefit from a spiritually meaningful trip, says Alice D. Domar, Ph.D., assistant professor of medicine at Harvard Medical School and director of the Mind/Body Center for Women's Health at Beth Israel Deaconess Medical Center in Boston.

"Spiritual vacations offer an opportunity to learn skills that you can apply to everyday life," Domar says. "On a regular vacation, sometimes the tendency is to eat and drink too much. You're always busy sightseeing or shopping. But when you go on a trip like this, you're in a lovely environment with fresh air and healthy food, and you're getting lots of sleep. You're also forcing yourself to spend time looking at your inner self."

Moreover, she says, spiritual vacations offer people an opportunity to enhance their health by learning valuable relaxation skills. "It's especially good when you're on a tour or at a retreat with teachers who can guide you as you learn and practice. It's a little like having a therapist on vacation with you."

Domar says spiritual travel is on the rise, and industry statistics back her up. When it opened 20 years ago, only a handful of spiritual seekers visited Omega Institute, a holistic retreat in Rhinebeck, New York. Today the center attracts an annual 12,000 guests, who take three- to seven-day workshops on a variety of spiritually based topics.

Sedona, Arizona, considered by some to be the metaphysical capital of the United States, also reports steady increases in visitors who immerse themselves in mineral-rich mud, shop for crystals in New Age stores and soak up energy from natural vortexes, which they believe radiate a rejuvenating electromagnetic force.

"Spiritual travel is definitely on the increase," says Nikki Harvey-Waring, manager of New Age Travel in Queensland, Australia. "I believe that people are looking to get away from the pressures of daily life. They're looking to have a meaningful experience instead of visiting the normal holiday areas."

Harvey-Waring is among the many tour operators who offer spiritual trips to India, Machu Picchu in Peru, Sedona, and Hawaii. Other popular destinations include Egypt, England's Stonehenge, Tibet, Nepal and the Bible lands of the Middle East.

Spiritual travel has always attracted the faithful. For centuries Muslims have trekked to the holy city of Mecca in Saudi Arabia. Chaucer's *Canterbury Tales*, moreover, revolves around a group of 14th-century Christian pilgrims.

What's new is that more people—who may not necessarily consider themselves to be traditionally religious—are opting to spend their leisure time discovering new ways to nourish their souls.

"All types of people come to Sedona," says Mark Goncalo, a tour guide and teacher of Arizona history at a community college near Phoenix. "But they all have one thing in common: They're all seeking something."

And many spiritual travelers find it, says Ellen Cayce, manager of A.R.E. Tours, a division of the Association for Research and Enlightenment in Virginia Beach, Virginia. A.R.E. transports believers to sites referred to by Edgar Cayce, the late "sleeping prophet," who gave hundreds of thousands of metaphysical readings while in a trance. Popular destinations include Egypt, Israel and India, says Ellen Cayce, Edgar's granddaughter by marriage.

"Our groups bond through meditation, dream sharing and inspirational focus as they travel," she says. "One of our goals is that our participants come to know themselves at deeper and more meaningful levels while seeing and experiencing the world."

Let Your Spirit Soar

Scores of tour operators offer a variety of vacations to metaphysical destinations around the world, where you can learn meditation and relaxation skills, study with shamans in tropical rain forests, climb ancient pyramids, or practice yoga on a mountain top.

Depending on the type of trip you take and the destination you choose, you can spend anywhere from a few hundred dollars to several thousand. Here are some organizations that can help you to plan your trip and get to know yourself better.

Mystical Journeys
Highlights: Healing ceremonies at vortex power centers in Inca "hot spots" such as Cusco and Machu Picchu. Tel. (800) 369-7842

Power Places Tours
Highlights: Pyramids of Egypt, mountain climbing in Tibet and Nepal, hiking through a Brazilian rain forest. Tel. (800) 234-8687

Myths and Mountains
Highlights: Trips to holy sites in South America and Asia. Tel. (800) 670-6984

A.R.E. Tours
Highlights: Metaphysical destinations cited by prophet Edgar Cayce. Tel. (888) 273-3339

> *Can't find the time for a full-fledged vacation? Consider devoting just a day or two to exercising your spiritual muscles. Spas, retreats and wellness centers can help to heal body, mind and spirit, as well as teach you how to take responsibility for your health and well-being.*

Ah, Spa...
Removing yourself from workaday concerns can help you to get in touch with your higher self. But you needn't take off from work for a week or break the bank to break your routine. Consider a retreat. Just a day or two is all you need.

Many monasteries welcome weekend guests. This is a great way to remove yourself from the busy world and reflect on life. If you can't find a monastery in your area, consider going on a solo camping trip. Build a campfire and watch the stars come out. Or simply set aside an afternoon to sit quietly in your bedroom.

"A retreat is simply a method to help us slow down," says David A. Cooper, author of *Silence, Simplicity and Solitude*. "Our own home has many advantages in terms of convenience, comfort, cost, timing and a sense of security."

You also may want to visit a spa. A full-body massage or aromatherapy treatment can do wonders for your body as well as your soul. Choose from a wide variety of soothing, uplifting therapies.

It used to be that spas were where the rich and famous went to shed pounds or stop drinking. Today, "Spas are evolving into the preventive medicine centers for the next century," says Diane Tegmeyer, author of *The Spa Lifestyle at Home.* "Spas are about getting a prescription for life."

Spa attendance, in fact, has been growing by leaps and bounds, according to the International Spa and Fitness Association.

Think of spas and retreats as "lifestyle universities," where participants learn about healthy foods and diet; spirituality and mind/body techniques; and traditional and alternative medicine. Then take that knowledge home with you and get to work on exercising your spirit!

Choosing a Retreat

With so many spas, retreats and wellness centers around the country, how do you choose one that's right for you? Here's a look at what some of the nation's top retreats have to offer.

Chopra Center at La Costa Resort & Spa

Deepak Chopra, who helped to mainstream Indian Ayurvedic medicine, offers anti-aging therapy; educational programs, with classes in nutrition, body types, meditation and herbal remedies; and research, which he uses to support his therapies.

Located in Carlsbad, CA. Tel. (800) 854-5000

Esalen Institute

This self-styled "emotional boot camp" is on 27 acres between the Pacific and the Santa Lucia mountains. Esalen is famous for its theater-based skits and workshops, which explore the mind/body connection via East/West philosophies and experimental techniques. There are also workshops on personal growth and holistic health, including shamanic healing, Gestalt therapy and neurolinguistics, and bodywork techniques including Rolfking, Feldenkrais and deep-tissue massage.

Located in Big Sur, CA. Tel. (831) 667-3000

Golden Door

Japanese-inspired architecture and gardens amid 350 acres of orchards and woodlands help guests to achieve a sense of serenity as they practice meditation, hatha yoga, and tai chi, among other therapies. Participants also are encouraged to explore creative pursuits such as music and crafts. In addition, you're provided with a complete spa wardrobe for use during your stay.

Located in Escondido, CA. Tel. (800) 424-0777

Kripalu Center for Yoga and Health

On 300 acres of forest and lakefront in the beautiful Berkshires, this spiritual sanctuary on the site of a former Jesuit seminary introduces guests to self-healing techniques for enhancing personal and spiritual growth. Classes ranges from yoga and meditation to breathwork and shiatsu. Guests also may enjoy meditation rooms, saunas, video lounges, and a private beach on Lake Mahkeenac.

Located in Lenox, MA. Tel. (800) 741-7353

Omega Institute for Holistic Studies

Founded in 1977, Omega offers myriad courses, ranging from yoga and meditative breathing to tai chi and dance therapy. When you're not in class, you're free to commune with 80 acres of forest, apple orchards, organic gardens and tranquil lakes. In addition, Omega offers treatments that range from aromatherapy, shiatsu and reflexology to therapeutic massage and sauna.

Located in Rhinebeck, NY. Tel. (800) 944-1001

The Peaks at Telluride

There's a 42,000-square-foot spa at this 10-story luxury mountain resort overlooking green foothills and rocky outcrops. Rejuvenation of mind, body and spirit is the center's goal. A personal spa concierge assists guests in creating a customized program of natural therapies. You'll also find workshops on astrology, breathwork, chakra clearing, homeopathy, therapeutic touch, Tibetan healing sounds, various types of massage, aromatherapy, hydrotherapy, reiki, reflexology, stress management, body wraps and scrubs, facials, salon services, cooking demonstrations, health lectures, journaling sessions.

Located in Telluride, CO. Tel. (800) 789-2220

Tassajara Zen Mountain Center

This working Zen monastery welcomes guests for summer workshops and retreats focusing on Zen philosophy, gardening and healthy cooking. You can meditate with the monks-or simply enjoy the breathtaking beauty of the countryside. The monastery also features a library, steam rooms, sun decks, swimming pool, sulfur springs and hiking trails.

Located in Carmel Valley, CA. Tel. (831) 659-2229

Spirit Action Plan

•**Go on a spiritual scavenger hunt**. Read books from various traditions, visit different churches, talk with friends about their attitudes and beliefs.

•**Turn off the TV**. Read a poem or listen to a recorded symphony.

•**Lose the news**. Try imposing a moratorium on news for one day a week. In this era of instant communications, we tend to suffer from information overload. Do you really need to know every detail about an earthquake in Albania?

•**Give of yourself.** Smile at a stranger at least once a day. Babysit for a friend. Cook dinner for a neighbor. Volunteer your skills.

•**Park it.** One of the easiest ways to center yourself is to go for a walk in the park. Take a deep breath and enjoy the scenery. Commune with a squirrel.

8. Fun

It's Fun to Feel Better

All work and no play doesn't just make you dull—it can make you sick. For a truly healthy lifestyle it's essential to have more than just a little fun. Enjoy yourself every day!

It's not just an old saying. Laughter may be the best medicine after all. Mounting research points to a strong link between health, longevity and the ability to enjoy life.

You've heard what laughter did for Norman Cousins. The longtime editor of the *Saturday Review* suffered from a crippling arthritic condition, but nursed himself back to health by chuckling at old tapes of *Candid Camera* television programs and Marx Brothers movies. Cousins claimed that just 10 minutes of good, old-fashioned belly laughing produced an "anesthetic" effect that gave him at least two hours of pain-free sleep.

"Modern science is beginning to confirm that this kind of laughter is not only enjoyable, it's also health-promoting," says David S. Sobel, M.D.

Nobody is suggesting that you morph into a couch potato, but sometimes watching TV is a good thing. In one study, people who enjoyed a tape of Lily Tomlin joking about the telephone company were less sensitive to pain than respondents who listened to an academic lecture. In another study, participants who watched a Richard Pryor tape produced elevated levels of antibodies in saliva, which help our bodies to fight against infections, such as colds.

That's because laughter appears to stimulate production of brain chemicals called catecholamines and endorphins. These affect the body's hormone levels, which ease pain, strengthen the immune system and contribute to feelings of joy.

Being able to laugh at the world around us helps our bodies to deal with stress and battle illness, says John Morreall, Ph.D., who has studied the effects of laughter on health. "The person who has a sense of humor is not just more relaxed in the face of potentially stressful situations but is more flexible in his approach."

Being more flexible may enable us to change our bodily responses when confronted with sickness. Several studies, for example, indicate that humor helps to boost immune-system functions.

Babies begin to laugh when they are just 10 weeks old; six weeks later, they're laughing, on average, about once an hour. Most grownups, however, let loose with a laugh only about 15 times a day.

"We learn to associate growing up with getting serious,'" says Sobel. "We are ordered to 'Wipe that smile off your face' and told that many events are no laughing matter."

But the ability to laugh is what makes us human. "Humor is, by far, the most significant behavior of the human mind," says Edward de Bono, M.D., an authority on the physiology of creativity.

Need a Lift?

Put more humor in your life. Every day presents us with opportunities to laugh at ourselves and the world around us. By doing so, you'll feel and look years younger. Here's how to lighten up:

•**Cultivate a sense of cosmic humor**. Look for the ridiculous, incongruous events that go on around you all the time.

•**Laugh 100 times a day**, recommends William F. Fry, Jr., M.D., emeritus associate clinical professor in the Department of Psychiatry at Stanford University School of Medicine. Laughter, he says, releases endorphins and boosts your immune system.

•**Start a humor library** of books, magazines, movies, cartoons.

Work at Having Fun

A quick infusion of light-heartedness can boost your energy levels and even improve cognitive processes, such as judgment, problem solving and decision making. Every day, in fact, we have myriad opportunities to exercise our sense of humor. A good place to start is at your job.

Most of us spend at least eight hours a day working for a living. But do you love what you do? Researchers are discovering that doing something you love can strengthen the immune system and help you to look and feel years younger.

10 Tips for Managing Job Stress

Feel like dumping dirt on your desk, strangling your supervisor? You're not alone. In recent years, employee rage has darkened workplaces around the country. Let's face it, holding down a job is serious business for most of us. After all, we have to earn money to survive. In addition, more than a few folks use their jobs to validate their self worth—and that can be dangerous. Don't let your job get the best of you. Learn to love your work. Here are some ways to beat back work-induced stress.

1. Take a break. Stretching, walking, meditating and other relaxation techniques can help at break time. Just stretching while you're listening to voice mail can help.

2. Take time for yourself. Don't work while you're having lunch. Don't allow coworkers to interrupt you when you're on your break.

3. Look for support. Make friends in the workplace with whom you can share feelings and concerns. But don't spend all your time complaining about the job. Avoid coworkers who do.

4. Meet with your supervisor. Talk about your job and performance at least once a year; every quarter or six months is even better.

5. Be assertive at work—not aggressive.

6. Manage your time. Leave your job at the office at the end of the day, even if your office is at home. Ask for a flexible schedule if your employer allows for one.

7. Pull the plug. Stay away from the Internet and cell phones during free time. Don't let new technology eradicate boundaries between your time and your employer's time.

8. Be creative. Come up with new ways to improve your job or the company's overall functioning.

9. Change your thinking. Try being positive about your job, if just for one day.

10. Know when to leave. If you hate your job and can't change it, get out. Being unemployed is better than working at a job you hate.

"Passion for work keeps you excited about what you are doing, and being excited about work helps keep you feeling vibrant," says workplace consultant Mildred Culp, Ph.D. "As most people get older they have to fight getting stale on the job. If they don't, the child within them may disappear. But if you create something in your work that causes passion, then you will always be alive."

Richard Bolles, author of the best-selling *What Color is Your Parachute?*, agrees. "Enthusiasm for work fuels the psyche and the spirit,. It's the feeling that you're eager to wake up in the morning and greet the day. It's the foundation for defining your purpose in life. Many people who retire die prematurely because they have no worthwhile definition of why they are still here on earth."

Loving your job may even help you to fend off heart disease, says Larry Dossy, M.D., author of *Healing Words*. A few years ago, researchers noticed that people were more apt to have heart attacks at about 9 a.m. on a Monday than any other time of the week.

"If you hate your job, you're going to be at much greater risk for Black Monday Syndrome," says Dossy. "Your attitude toward your work is critical. It's a huge predictor of heart disease."

Some researchers speculate that a good attitude on the job triggers the brain to release endorphins and other chemicals that fight disease and may even help to suppress tumor growth.

It's equally important to keep on smiling after you've punched that timeclock at the end of the day. Leave your worries at the door. Home, after all, is where the heart is, not where you continue to work.

Pack your personal life with fun. Enjoy your home and family. Studies show that married people live longer than those who are single. Don't have a family? Make one. Invite your next-door neighbor to dinner, volunteer at a local charity, go online and visit a chat room. Toss a ball to your dog. If you don't have a dog, get one, or a cat, or a hamster. Having pets can make a real difference in your health.

"Pets improve health because they help people to adapt, adjust and deal with changes," says Alan Entin, Ph.D., past president of the division of family psychology of the American Psychological Association.

Studies have shown, for example, that pet owners who suffered heart attacks were likely to enjoy five times the survival rate of patients who did not own pets, says cardiologist Stephen Sinatra, who runs the Heart and Longevity Center in Manchester, Connecticut. In addition, a pet's unconditional love gives its owner a sense of worth and responsibility.

Create Good Health

You'll also feel better if you take up a hobby or recreation. Sports and activities such as walking are wonderful ways to enhance your health.

Also consider creative endeavors to nurture body, mind and spirit.

Drawing helped Lucia Capacchione to recover from a debilitating collagen disease.

"I went inside myself and began drawing and writing my innermost feelings," says Capacchione, who described her healing journey in *The Picture of Health*. "Just expressing my feelings in the moment was liberating in itself. The fear, anger and grief that had been buried so long all came out on paper. A few months later I was completely cured."

OK, you're no Picasso. But you do know how to write, don't you? Jotting down your feelings in a journal may the write medicine for you. Not only that, writing can be loads of fun.

Researchers at North Dakota State University in Fargo presented pens to 112 patients with asthma and rheumatoid arthritis. They asked some of the patients to write about the most stressful experiences of their lives. The remaining patients were instructed to write about subjects that held no meaning for them.

Four months later, the researchers noted dramatic improvements in nearly half of the patients who had expressed powerful emotions. But the patients who wrote about emotionally neutral topics reported far fewer improvements.

"These gains were beyond those attributed to the standard medical care that the participants were receiving," says Joshua M. Smyth, Ph.D., who headed up the research team.

Pet a Pussy

Simply petting an animal causes blood pressure to drop in most people, says Alan Beck, director of the Center for the Human-Animal Bond at Purdue University. Owning a pet offers even more health benefits.

Researchers at the State University of New York in Buffalo examined the effects of pet ownership on 48 stockbrokers who were taking medication for hypertension. The study found that the 24 participants who were given a pet demonstrated a significantly greater reduction in high blood pressure than those who had no pets.

What caused the gains? Was it mind over matter? Yes and no, says David Spiegel, M.D., of Stanford University School of Medicine in Palo Alto, California. "It's not simply mind over matter," he says. "But it is clear that mind matters."

The key appears to be expressing your innermost feelings. Patients improved only after writing about events that had a powerful impact on their lives. As they remembered those painful moments, Smyth says, they became visibly upset and experienced changes in heart rate and blood pressure. Moreover, Smyth speculates, it may be that getting out bottled-up feelings helps to boost the body's disease-fighting immune system.

"Studies show that even limited interventions to improve management of stress have lasting physical effects," says Spiegel. "It's important to combine this type of intervention with other forms of more traditional medical care."

How to Keep a Diary

Intimidated by a blank piece of paper? You're not alone. Many people are frightened by the prospect of recording their feelings, says Natalie Goldberg, who writes in her journal as a form of meditation.

But anyone can keep a diary, says Goldberg, author of *Writing Down the Bones: Freeing the Writer Within*. "There is no logical A-to-B-to-C way to become a writer," she says. "It's not a linear process."

In other words, there is no right or wrong way to do it. Here are some tips to help you get started:

•Buy a notebook that appeals to you. Does it have an attractive cover? Pick it up and flip through the pages. Do you like the way it feels?
•Try to write at the same time each day. That way writing will become a habit. Write early in the morning before you go to work or pack the kids off to school. Or record your thoughts at night, before you go to bed.
•Don't think you have to be profound. Leave that to Norman Mailer. "All the journal requires is the most basic writing ability and the desire to articulate the journey," says Christina Baldwin, author of *Life's Companion: Journal Writing as a Spiritual Quest*.
•Remember that nobody's perfect. "It doesn't matter if you spell correctly, write fancifully, go into expansive detail, or leave only brief notations to aid recall," Baldwin says. "Whatever works works."
•Let it flow. Simply spill out your thoughts in what writers call "stream of consciousness." To start, Baldwin advises, pick an object—any object—and observe it for a moment. "Then allow your thoughts to free-associate. Jot them down as they occur."

•Write what you feel. Remember, this is your diary and you can say whatever you want. "The journal," Baldwin says, "is a private document."

Other Paths to Creative Expression

There are hundreds of ways to express creativity. Take up needlepoint. Learn how to change the oil in your car. Teach yourself to play guitar—or simply listen to music. Several studies show that music not only soothes the savage breast, it also:

•Helps stroke victims to recover faster. Researchers at Colorado State University say patients recovering from strokes found it easier to relearn to walk if they listened to music every day. Scottish scientists, moreover, have discovered that music can reduce depression and boost the spirits of stroke victims.

•Cuts pain and help us to heal faster. A Michigan cardiologist played music 20 minutes a day for patients recovering from heart surgery. The music did as a much as drugs to reduce pain, and the patients went home four days early.

•Makes us smarter! In 1993 researchers at the University of California, Irvine, concluded that listening to Mozart before taking an IQ test boosted scores by about nine points.

"I regard music therapy as a tool of great power," says Oliver Sacks, M.D, whose work with neurological patients inspired the move *Awakenings*. "Music has a unique capacity to organize and reorganize cerebral functioning when it has been damaged."

Researchers know that listening to music directly influences pulse rate, blood pressure and electrical activity of muscles. Now neurologists think that music may help to build and strengthen connections among nerve cells.

As a result, more hospitals are prescribing music to alleviate pain, boost moods, promote relaxation and induce sleep. Experts say that music therapy is effective for children and adults alike. And music can be used to treat a wide range of conditions, including mental illness, learning disabilities, Alzheimer's and other brain diseases; physical disabilities, and acute and chronic pain.

"Music can assist in the physical healing process in several ways," says Steven Halpern, a California composer of music to help people to relax, heal emotional and physical problems and break bad habits. "Music can help the body to heal itself, which the body does effectively in a state of deep relaxation."

It's never too early to develop an appreciation of music, therapists say. In fact, music can help to bring us into the world. Texas therapists, for example, found that women who listened to music while in labor needed less anesthesia than women who didn't.

Louisiana researchers concluded in 1995 that listening to lullabies enabled premature babies to go home earlier than infants who were not exposed to music. And Deforia Lane, a music therapist at University Hospitals in Cleveland, has shown that music even boosts immune function in children. "It's a mystery," Lane says, "but it works."

A great place to listen to music is the bedroom. Turn on the CD player and then turn on each other. Good sex is good for your health.

Cuddle Up

There's a biological reason for sex—it's the way we keep the species going. But sex also is a lot of fun, and you can't have too much fun in your life, right?

You know that "glow" you get after making love? Scientists attribute it to endorphins, the feel-good chemicals that are released into the brain after sex. Endorphins create a sense of euphoria and ease stress. What's more, endorphins released by sex can help us to heal.

Medical researchers say that regular doses of sex soothe chronic aches and pains, spur creativity, and rev up energy. In fact, says "sexpert" Helen S. Kaplan, M.D., Ph.D., intimacy can bolster your immune system and protect you from developing age-related diseases.

Researchers have found a key relationship between sexual energy and two biological cycles: the 24-hour circadian rhythm and the 60- to 90-minute ultradian rhythm. Sexually satisfied couples tend to have overall activity patterns, appetite, need for diversion and sexual rhythms occurring in synchronicity.

So get in synch with someone you love and you'll feel years younger. "Anything that makes you feel good, alive and physically excited will make you feel more youthful," says Lonnie Barbach, Ph.D., a sex therapist and psychologist in San Francisco.

Intimacy can add youthful years to your life, says "sexpert" Helen Kaplan. Where do you start? Here are some simple steps you can take to help you develop a more intimate relationship with your lover:

•Kiss your partner whenever you leave or arrive, using the sensory power of touch to realign your energy cycles.

- Slow down the pace of your evening meal. Enjoy each other's company. Talk.
- Go for an early morning or evening stroll together.
- Spend time fixing meals together, doing dishes or puttering around the garden.
- Sit together quietly, holding hands.
- Listen to music you both enjoy.
- Sip a cup of tea or a glass of wine together.
- Share a warm bath or gentle rhythmic massage for 15 minutes before sex.
- Stretch out on the sofa and hold each other.
- Turn sex play into love play. "Touch may be the most powerful socio-biological signal of all," says psychobiologist Ernest Lawrence Rossi, Ph.D. "When we are touched gently and rhythmyically, our brains release the feel-good messenger chemicals called beta-endorphins and we slip into the psychologically receptive state where we're open to increased intimacy."
- Fantasize. Anticipate sex. Let your imagination soar.
- Create an atmosphere of intimate safety and trust for you and your partner.
- Relax. Let go of all distractions and worries.
- Share your favorite sensations. Let your partner know what turns you on.
- Have a hot date once a week even if you've been married for 30 years or more.
- Listen. "By learning to listen to a woman's feelings, a man can effectively shower her with caring, understanding, respect, devotion, validation and reassurance," says best-selling relationship author John Gray, Ph.D.
- Make eye contact. "Eyes speak more profoundly than language the tenor of relatedness," says psychologist Ruthellen Josselson, Ph.D. "They express surely and absolutely how much and in what way we matter to the other."
- Snuggle. "Holding contains the invisible threads that ties us to our existence," says Josselson. "From the first moments of our life to the last we need to be held—or we fall."
- Laugh more. A study at Tel Aviv University in Israel concluded that 70 percent of a married couple's satisfaction may depend in some way on humor.

Fun Action Plan

•**Remember to laugh**. In our hectic world, it ís easy to forget. Before you go to sleep, ask yourself: How many times did I laugh today? Surely you can come up with one funny thing that happened to you.

•**Adopt a pet**. Pick out a puppy or a kitten at the pound. The love you get back will be worth every minute of the effort it takes to care for the animal.

•**Introduce yourself to your inner child**. Buy a coloring book at the grocery store—or a bottle of bubble liquid or a ball and jacks. You enjoyed those things once. Who says you have to stop just because you got big?

•**Pull the plug**. Who wants to live in a world without an Internet or cell phones? But that doesn ít mean you have to be ìavailableî 24 hours a day. Take a break.

•**Learn to love your job.** If you can ít, quit and find another one you do like.

9. Home

Clean up Your Act

When was the last time you vacuumed under the sofa? Keeping a clean house isn't just cosmetic. You may not realize it, but your dirty home may be killing you.

You're eating foods that are good for you. You're exercising. You've tried meditating and breathing exercises to relax. You're getting a good night's sleep and you're remembering to put a little fun in your life. You're stronger now, but you're still not feeling up to par. Have you looked under your sink?

If you're like most Americans, the cabinets and shelves in your kitchen, bathroom and garage are crammed with chemicals: disinfectants, furniture polishes, glass cleaners, shampoos, conditioners, lotions, paints and pesticides. Many of these common commodities contain poisons ranging from formaldehyde and petroleum distillates to hydrochloric acid, and we're exposing ourselves to them every day.

Mounting research indicates that many common illnesses, from respiratory infections to arthritis, are caused or worsened by exposure to environmental toxins. The really frightening part is that most of us are unaware of the dangers lurking behind our doors.

"Even if you follow the directions, there are real health risks of using common household products," says author and natural healing advocate

Why take a chance on potentially risky household chemicals? Dump 'em.

James Balch, M.D. "More and more, I'm seeing patients who complain of a variety of chronic ailments: irritating allergies; nagging coughs; persistent colds; aching muscles, and other flu-like symptoms, and these may be caused by the toxins in their homes."

Home Sweet Home?

The houses that we live in may be just as toxic as a public dump. Don't believe it? Here are the facts:

• In large numbers of U.S. homes, chemical levels are 70 times higher inside than outdoors, according to a five-year study by the federal Environmental Protection Agency.
• In 1988 more than 9,000 people sought emergency room treatment for injuries caused by household bleaches, reports the U.S. Consumer Product Safety Commission. More than 60 percent of patients were under 5 years old.
• Indoor air pollution is responsible for more deaths around the globe than outdoor air—even in the most contaminated cities, such as Bangkok and Mexico City, according to the World Health Organization.

Even more disturbing is that indoor toxins don't disappear after we use them. Fumes linger in our homes and we breathe them again and again. What's more, no one—not even the government—knows what effect such chemicals are having on our bodies.

We have no information, for example, on toxic effects of 79 percent of more than 48,500 synthetic chemicals listed by the EPA. Fewer than one-fifth of all common chemicals have been tested for acute dangers; fewer than one-tenth for chronic, reproductive or mutagenic effects.

Step outside and you're confronted with more potential chemical dangers. Your garage, patio and backyard may harbor a number of highly poisonous substances: paint; paint thinner, benzene, kerosene, mineral spirits, turpentine, motor oil and gasoline. Charcoal lighter fluid contains petroleum distillates, which are highly flammable, and some contain benzene, a known carcinogen.

Also consider that in more than 34,000 consumer products are 1,400 pesticides, herbicides and fungicides, alone or combined with solvents and other toxic substances. Several new studies indicate that use of pesticides in the home is directly related to increasing incidences of childhood cancers. Is it any wonder that health-care costs are skyrocketing?

Take a Tour of Your Home

You're probably not aware of the potential dangers lurking in every room of your home. Let's take a walk-through of an average house and peek inside the cupboards. Here's what we're likely to find.

Kitchen

Glass cleaners. They contain ammonia, which may irritate eyes, cause headaches and damage lungs.

Disinfectants. Common chemical ingredients are phenol and cresol, which are corrosive and may cause diarrhea, fainting, dizziness and kidney and liver damage.

Laundry Room

Fabric softeners. Some people are allergic to the chemical fragrances added to these products.

Spray starch. Ingredients may include formaldehyde, phenol and pentachlorophenol. In addition, any aerosol product may irritate the lungs.

Detergent. Petrochemicals form the basis of many such products, which also may contain irritating fragrances. In addition, most detergents contain phosphates, which build up in streams and lakes, depleting the oxygen that fish need to survive. Some detergents also contain hazardous naphthalene or phenol.

Chlorine bleach. If mixed with ammonia, the hypochlorite in this product produces toxic chloramine gas. Short-term exposure may cause mild asthmatic symptoms or more serious respiratory problems.

Family Rooms

Furniture. If you're like many Americans, most of your furniture is not made of solid wood but of processed pressed wood that emits formaldehyde and other chemicals.

Carpets. Synthetic fibers usually are treated with pesticides and fungicides. In the latex backing may be a chemical called 4-phenylcyclohexene, which is thought to be one of the chemicals responsible for "sick building syndrome."

Floor polish. Skin discoloration, shallow breathing, vomiting, birth defects and cancer are among possible conditions caused by nitrobenzene, an ingredient of many floor polishes.

Carpet cleaners/spot removers. Perchloroethylene and 1-1-1 trichloroethane solvents are among the toxins in these products. The chemicals may cause liver and kidney damage if ingested; perchloroethylene causes cancer in animals and may cause cancer in humans.

Metal polishes. Often they're based on petroleum distillates. Short-term exposure may cause your vision to cloud; longer exposure may damage the nervous system, skin, kidneys, and eyes.

Bedroom

Sheets. Your "wrinkle resistant," no-iron sheets, linens, curtains and pajamas probably have been treated with a formaldehyde resin. Be wary of polyester/cotton blends marketed as "permanent press" or "easy care."

Mothballs. Naphthalene, found in mothballs, is a suspected carcinogen that may damage eyes, blood, liver, kidneys, skin, and the central nervous system; paradichlorobenzene, another ingredient, may harm the central nervous system, liver, and kidneys.

Bathrooms

Shampoo. Here's what you may be putting in your hair: formaldehyde, glycols, nitrates/nitrosamines and sulfur compounds.

Hair spray. Butane propellants, carcinogenic methylene chloride and formaldehyde resins are just some of the chemicals often found in these products..

Antiperspirant deodorants. They're packed with aerosol propellants, ammonia, formaldehyde, triclosan and aluminum chlorhydrate.

Lotions, creams and moisturizers. List among their ingredients glycols and potentially irritating artificial fragrances and colors.

Toilet bowl cleaners. You're likely to find hydrochloric acid and sodium acid sulfate, which may burn skin or cause vomiting, diarrhea and stomach burns if swallowed. These chemicals also may cause blindness if accidentally splashed in eyes.

Garage, Patio, Backyard

Paint thinners. Often they contain clorinated alipathic and aromatic hydrocarbons, which may cause liver and kidney damage. They also contain ketones and toluene, as does wood putty. These may cause respiratory ailments. Toluene is especially toxic and may cause skin, liver and central nervous-system and reproductive-system damage.

Oil-based paints. Ingredients include mineral spirits, which irritate skin, eye, nose, throat and lungs. High concentrations may cause nervous-system damage, unconsciousness and death.

Gasoline/motor oils. These contain petroleum hydrocarbons and benzene, which have been associated with skin and lung cancers.

Where Did They Come From?

A hundred years ago no one worried about toxic homes. Back then folks lived a simpler, safer life. They used plain old soap, vinegar, baking soda, ammonia, borax and cornstarch to lift out spots and stains, deodorize, polish, disinfect, scrub, repel pests, clean pets, wash clothes and kids. They didn't need dangerous, expensive fertilizers to feed their tomatoes; they nourished vegetable gardens with organic compost made from kitchen scraps.

If you bought a table or bookcase, it was made of real wood, not processed sawdust. You kept that wood clean by polishing it with natural oils, not chemical sprays. The rugs and carpets on floors were produced from sheep-sheared wool and cotton, not synthetic fibers. Builders, moreover, insulated homes not by lining them with toxic materials but by making thicker walls.

The chemical industry put an end to all that. It evolved, ostensibly, to make our lives easier. It's done that on some levels, but it's also opened up a whole new can of worms. Since World War II, manufacturers have introduced more than 70,000 synthetic chemicals to American consumers. The United States alone produces 250 billion pounds of synthetic chemicals each year.

Many of these chemicals are in common household products. We use them every day to wash our bodies and our floors, clean our clothes and our children's bedrooms. We brush our teeth with them, wash our hair with them, moisturize our skin with them. In addition, 75 percent of U.S. households use chemicals to kill pests and eradicate weeds.

And we never give them a second thought.

It's never too late to clean up your home. Reduce or eliminate health risks by making thoughtful purchases at the supermarket and substituting safe products for harmful ones.

Heal Your Sick Home

Because we spend so much of our time indoors—90 percent of our time, according to the EPA—it is imperative that we clean up our homes. Defending your home against toxins may seem overwhelming at first. But you have many tools at your disposal to keep your home sparkling and make it the safe haven you always thought it was.

Start by throwing out all those toxic products under the sink. Read labels on products you buy. Avoid those with hazardous ingredients. In most cases, you don't even need special products to clean your home. A handful of common, natural products will keep your house sparkling, while promoting good health.

Baking Soda. It's probably in your kitchen right now. Put it to better uses. Baking soda is perfect for removing odors from the refrigerator, carpets and drains. It softens fabrics and removes stains. Baking soda can soften "hard" water and makes for a relaxing bath-time soak. You can even use it as an underarm deodorant and toothpaste.

In addition, use it as a remedy for heartburn, to scrub cabinets, pots and pans without scratching, even to put out grease fires.

Borax. Mix this mineral with sugar to attract and kill cockroaches. Borax also deodorizes, attacks mildew and mold, boosts the cleansing power of soap or detergent and removes stains.

Cornstarch. A thin paste of cornstarch and water will lift stains from carpets and rugs. Also use cornstarch to clean windows and polish furniture.

Lemon Juice. Use it in sunlight to lighten fabrics like bleach. Lemon juice also is great to deodorize, clean glass, and remove stains from aluminum, clothes and porcelain.

Mineral Oil. It's a safe, natural furniture polish and floor wax.

Soap. Natural castile soap makes a great body cleanser and shampoo. Soaps made from olive oil are good for your skin.

Steel Wool. Tackle almost any stain with steel wool dipped in borax. This abrasive is tough enough to remove even rust and stubborn food stains and to scrub barbecue grills.

Vinegar. This may be the most important product you keep in your home. Buy it by the gallon. It does almost everything. Use vinegar to clean brick and stone, get rid of the metallic taste in coffeepots and clean windows with no streaks. It also dissolves mineral deposits and grease, removes soap, mildew and was buildup, deodorizes fabrics and polishes some metals.

Plants don't just make a room look prettier. They help to heal sick rooms, too. Plants remove carbon dioxide from the air, along with chemicals such as formaldehyde.

Just two potted plants for every 100 feet of floor space can help to clean the air in your home.

Recipes for a Healthy Home

It's easy to keep your home clean and naturally healthy. Next time you're tempted to reach for a chemical product, try whipping up one of these:

Cleaners

Air freshener: Simmer cinnamon and cloves in apple juice. Put sliced lemons in your garbage disposal. Make potpourri from dried lemon and orange peels. Or simply open windows and doors.

All-purpose cleaner: Dissolve 4 tbs. baking soda in 1 quart of warm water or mix equal parts of vinegar and salt.

Detergent: There's nothing wrong with good old soap. Soap doesn't contain phosphates, fragrances or harsh chemicals. One-half to three-quarters of a cup of baking soda will leave clothes soft and fresh-smelling. Hand-wash silks and wools with mild soap or a protein-based shampoo. For synthetic fabrics and blends (including most no-iron fabrics) try biodegradable detergents from natural-food stores. Add a cup of vinegar to the wash to help keep colors bright, but don't use vinegar if you are using bleach or you may end up producing hazardous fumes.

Disinfectant: Disinfect and deodorize by mixing 1/2 cup borax with 1 gallon hot water, or simply clean with soap and hot water.

Drain cleaner: Open clogged drains by pouring 1/2 cup baking soda down the drain, followed by 1/2 cup white vinegar.

Floor polish: . For painted wooden floors, mix 1 tsp. baking soda with 1 gallon hot water. For brick and stone tiles, use 1 cup white vinegar with 1 gallon water, and rinse with clear water. For linoleum add a capful of baby oil to the water to bring back the shine. For wood floors apply a thin coat of equal parts oil and vinegar, and rub in well.

Add a few drops of vinegar to cleaning water to remove soap traces.

Glass cleaner: Your windows will shine if you use a solution of vinegar and water; cornstarch, vinegar and water; or lemon juice and water. Wipe with newspaper, unless you are sensitive to the inks in newsprint.

Metal cleaner: Clean stainless steel with undiluted white vinegar. Make a natural scouring powder form baking soda or table salt. Clean tarnished copper by boiling the piece in a pot of water with 1 tbs. salt and 1 cup white vinegar, or try mixtures of salt, vinegar, baking soda, or lemon juice. Clean gold with toothpaste. Pewter will come back to shiny new with a paste of salt, vinegar and flour. Silver may be polished by boiling it in a pan lined with aluminum foil and filled with water to which a teaspoon each of baking soda and salt have been added. Clean aluminum with a paste of cream of tartar and water. Brass shines up as bright as new with a soft cloth dipped in a lemon/baking soda or vinegar/salt solution. Polish chrome with baby oil, vinegar, or the shiny side of aluminum foil.

Oven cleaner: Steel wool and baking soda will get out the toughest stains.

Tile cleaner: Rinse with vinegar; then scrub with baking soda.

Toilet cleaner: Baking soda and vinegar, or borax and lemon juice work well to get out stubborn stains, use gloves and clean with baking soda and vinegar, or borax and lemon juice.

Cosmetics

Astringent/after shave: Witch hazel is a natural astringent that's good for your skin.

Conditioner: Chamomile tea is great for blondes; a tea made from sage and rosemary brings out highlights in brunettes. Or simply rinse hair with diluted vinegar.

Deodorant: Many people report success using baking soda, white clay or deodorant crystals.

Perfume: Essential oils are safe and effective.

Skin moisturizer/conditioner: Head for the kitchen. Treat your skin to natural moisturizers, such as egg yolks, milk, yogurt, safflower or olive oils.

Soap: Castile and olive oil-based soaps are natural and safe.

Shampoo: Good old soap works fine. Afterward, rinse with a natural conditioner.

Toothpaste: Before toothpaste was invented folks brushed their teeth with baking soda and salt.

Pesticides

Ants: Sprinkle powdered red chili pepper, paprika, dried peppermint, or borax where ants are entering the home.

Clean Your Insides

It's important to clean your body of toxins while you're getting your home naturally healthy, says James Balch, M.D. To help your body cleanse itself of toxins, here are some vitamins and supplements you may consider taking:

•**Vitamin C**: Ascorbic acid gives your whole system a boost.

•**Chlorella**: This helps your body to get rid of heavy metals in pollution.

•**Alpha lipoic acid**. This nutrient raises glutathione, which cleanses the body of toxins.

•**Milk thistle**: This herb also raises glutathione and helps the liver to detoxify your system.

•**Multivitamins and minerals**. Many help your body to produce toxin-removing enzymes.

Fleas: Feed your pets brewer's yeast. Not only will kit keep fleas at bay, it's rich in B vitamins and will give your pet bright eyes and a shiny coat.

Garden pests: Soapy water kills many of them.

Mice/rats: Close up holes in walls and keep storage spaces orderly. Tightly cover garbage cans. To catch rodents, take a tip from nature: Get a cat.

Moths: Make your own moth-repelling sachets of lavender, cedar chips or dried tobacco. Air clothes well in the sun; store in airtight containers with sachets.

Roaches: Mix 3 parts borax, 2 parts sugar and 4 parts flour. Spread over infested area. Repeat after four days and again after two weeks.

Termites: Any wooden parts of the house should be at least 18 inches off the ground; subterranean termites cannot tolerate exposure to air and light.

Home Healthy

We've begun a new century in a new millennium. Isn't it time we began to change our lives for the better? Make your home a natural home. You'll breathe a lot easier.

Home Action Plan

•**Trash the toxins**. Get rid of all those chemicals you use to clean your house and body.

•**Make your own**. Itís easy—and fun—to come up with safe, inexpensive substitutes for cleaners and cosmetics. Youíll feel better, your house will smell better and the world will be a better place for your kids.

•**Open your windows**. Air out the house from time to time.

•**Pot a plant**. Plants produce oxygen. Putting one in the living room is one of the easiest ways to clean your environment.

•**Scrub your insides**. Ask your doctor about herbs and supplements that may help to detoxify your body. Milk thistle, for example, helps your liver to get rid of poisons.

---

10. Staying Healthy

Keep up The Good Work!

You've worked long and hard to achieve a higher level of health. Don't let it all slip away. Stay on top of your game, maintain your goals and enjoy good health—now and forever!

You wouldn't neglect to take your car to the garage for periodic tuneups. Neither should you fail to take your body, mind and spirit in for a checkup from time to time.

It goes without saying that you need to see your doctor and dentist regularly. You don't need anyone to tell you that (anymore than you need for Burger King to warn on cups—in five languages, no less—that coffee tends to be hot.)

In today's HMO-regulated medical world, however, doctors aren't likely to give you all of the attention you need and deserve. You're lucky, in fact, if your doctor spends five minutes with you.

Take responsibility for your health. A number of alternative or complementary medical therapies, from acupuncture to hypnosis, may help you to maintain that level of health you've spent so much time attaining.

Yes, alternative medicine can be costly. A single acupuncture session may set you back fifty dollars or more. Save that money you might have spent at Burger King and put it in a "complementary medicine fund." Don't fail as well to check with your insurance plan. More insurers are reaching the conclusion (finally) that prevention is indeed the best cure.

More doctors also are coming to realize that western medicine does not hold all of the answers. China certainly could not have produced its teeming population if medicine there (which seems so strange to us) was not effective.

Healers long have relied on natural therapies to prevent and cure any number of illnesses. You'll need trained practitioners to provide some of these therapies. Others are safe enough for you to practice in the privacy of your home.

Have you ever considered trying acupuncture? More than 1 million Americans use acupuncture to treat ailments from headaches and stomach disorders to arthritis and stroke. Acupressure, a related technique, may be practiced at home.

On Pins & Needles

Acupuncture no longer is considered "weird." The ancient Chinese therapy, in fact, has become a growing business in the United States, employing more than 6,500 practitioners. In addition, more than 3,000 medical doctors and osteopaths in this country have attended acupuncture courses and incorporated the treatment in their practices.

"Acupuncture is definitely the next major area of interest" for the health-care industry, says healthcare consultant John Weeks.

Even the National Institutes of Health has recommended that doctors adopt acupuncture as a standard medical procedure. Acupuncture, says the NIH, is effective at treating a variety of medical conditions and has far fewer side effects than some conventional therapies. In particular, NIH says, acupuncture is a safe, reliable treatment for nausea associated with pregnancy and cancer chemotherapy, pain following dental surgery, and chronic problems such as low backache and asthma.

Developed in China more than 2,000 years ago, acupuncture involves placement of ultra-thin needles in the skin along specific meridians, or channels, through which *chi*—the body's life force—is believed to flow. There are 12 major acupuncture channels, and acupuncturists say that each is connected to an organ or body system. Therapists believe that they can stimulate the body's energy flow by manipulating the channels with needles.

Other forms of manipulation may be used as well. Some acupuncturists burn a stimulating herb called moxa (mugwort, or *Artemisia vulgaris*) above the treatment point. Another technique called "cupping" uses a glass or bamboo cup to create suction on the skin above a painful muscle or acupuncture point. Acupuncturists also may use electrostimulation, ultrasound waves, or laser beams. In addition, Chinese researchers have experimented with sonar rays and injections of water or steroids in acupuncture points.

Acupressure, a related therapy, is easy to perform on yourself. No needles are required. Instead, you use your fingers to press meridians and redirect your life force. Check out an acupressure book from the library and try it for yourself.

By manipulating chi, clinicians believe, you can alleviate many symptoms and cure some illnesses. The World Health Organization, in fact, cites more than 100 illnesses that appear to respond well to acupuncture.

"Acupuncture does work well to relieve many types of pain," says Barrie R. Cassileth, Ph.D., author of *The Alternative Medicine Handbook: The Complete Reference Guide to Alternative and Complementary Therapies*. Among conditions that respond well to the therapy, Cassileth says, are arthritis, premenstrual syndrome, chronic pain, and withdrawal symptoms associated with alcoholism, drug addiction and smoking.

But, Cassileth adds, "Just how it works remains unknown, and the existence of meridians remains unproven."

Nonetheless, there is considerable scientific evidence that acupuncture spurs release of natural pain-relieving substances in the body, such as endorphins, as well as messenger chemicals and hormones in the nervous system.

Your Body is a Battery

Several studies have measured the galvanic skin response of meridians and acupuncture points on the body. The studies suggest that these areas have a higher rate of electrical conductance than other parts of the body.

In the 1970s NIH researchers concluded that electrical currents do flow along the ancient Chinese meridians. Acupuncture points, they theorized, act as "amplifiers" to boost the body's electrical signals.

Although acupuncture long has been revered in China and other Asian countries, the treatment took a while to catch on in the West. Yao W. Lee, a doctor of Oriental Medicine with offices in Boca Raton and Fort Lauderdale, Florida, says he encountered considerable skepticism from conventional physicians in 1972, after he opened one of the first acupuncture clinics in the United States.

"Back then there was a lot of resistance," Lee recalls. "I was a pioneer in acupuncture and many of my patients told me their doctors told them not to do it."

Today, health practitioners such as Janet Konefal, maintain that the public interest in acupuncture "has opened the door for those in the medical field to step forward." At the University of Miami's Center for Complementary Medicine, where Konefal practices, doctors employ acupuncture to treat cancer, drug addiction and Parkinson's disease. "Physicians," she says, "are definitely warming up to acupuncture."

A Pound of Seal Penis, Please

Imagine walking out of Walgreen's with the dried penis of a seal. In China it's not unusual for people to do just that after visiting a traditional Chinese pharmacy.

Most Americans are unlikely to ask their pharmacists for the livers and kidneys of a gecko, but more of us are turning to Chinese herbs in an effort to heal ourselves naturally.

Because Chinese remedies are tailored to individual needs, it's best to see a doctor of Oriental medicine if you have a health problem. But there are many "tonic" herbs that you can safely consume to prevent illnesses and strengthen your system. Two you probably already know:

•**Angelica** (*Angelica sinensis*). Known in China as *dong quai*, angelica has been used extensively to treat menstrual-cycle disorders and symptoms of menopause.

•**Astragalus** (*Astragalus membranaceus*). This root is renowned for its ability to simulate the immune system and speed healing. Chinese doctors also recommend astragalus to treat weakness and excessive sweating.

Scientists in Hong Kong and other Chinese cities are making rapid advances in herbal medicine.

"We are studying herbs to treat cancer, heart disease, chronic fatigue syndrome, diabetes, and even AIDS," says Yang Wei Yi, a professor and herbal researcher at Hong Kong Baptist University.

Yang has experimented with ginseng (*Panax ginseng)* and magnolia bark (*Cortex magnoliae officinalis*), to treat the baffling Chronic Fatigue Syndrome, which incapacitates many of its victims as it drains them of energy.

"Western medicine can do very little to treat this condition," he says. "But we have discovered that many Chinese herbs can improve the immune system and regulate a number of physiological functions."

When it comes to natural therapies, China doesn't hold a monopoly. Americans also are discovering other techniques from Asia. Ayurvedic medicine from India is becoming increasingly popular with medically adventurous consumers.

There's more to India than curries. Ayurveda, an ancient healing system, appeals to many people searching for good health.

Ancient Healing

More than 5,000 years ago, healers in India devised a simple program of diet, exercise and meditation called Ayurveda. Today, thanks to endorsements by pop-doc superstars like Deepak Chopra, M.D., Americans are embracing the ancient healing regimen by the droves.

Ayurveda may be mankind's oldest form of mind-body medicine. "It was the Vedic seers who first recognized the unified field, now described by quantum physicists," says Nancy Lonsdorf, M.D., coauthor of *A Woman's Best Medicine: Health, Happiness and Long Life Through Ayur-veda*. "These healers first understood the science of the integration of human consciousness and the material world."

Ayurveda usually is translated as "the science of life," says Deepak Chopra, M.D., author of *Perfect Health: The Complete Mind/Body Guide*

Ayurveda's concept is simple, explains Chopra, a U.S.-trained physician who blends western medical techniques with Ayurvedic therapies. "The guiding principle of Ayurveda is that the mind exerts the deepest influence on the body. Freedom from sickness depends upon our contacting our awareness and bringing it into balance."

Vasant Lad, author of *The Complete Book of Ayurvedic Home Remedies*, calls Ayurveda "a science of self-healing. Ayurveda encompasses diet and nutrition, lifestyle, exercise, rest and relaxation, meditation, breathing exercises and medicinal herbs, along with cleansing and rejuvenation programs for healing body, mind and spirit."

Ayurvedic therapies are tailored to specific body types and lifestyles, Lad says. "According to Ayurveda, health is a perfect state of balance among the body's three fundamental energies or *doshas* (vata, pitta, kapha) and an equally vital balance among body, mind and the soul, or consciousness."

What's Your Dosha?

Don't know your dosha? Take a look at the characteristics for each and determine the one that suites you best.

Vata
Influence: Vata is the energy of movement.

Physical: Vata people tend to be small or underweight, with light, flexible bodies and cold, dry skin. They have less strength and stamina than others. Because they often suffer from poor circulation, they may be troubled by cold hands and feet. Vatas walk fast and always seem to be in a hurry. They may be attracted to jogging, jumping and other forms of physical exercise, but they tire easily. Vatas also may suffer from insomnia or interrupted sleep.

Emotional: Vatas may experience mood swings, and they have a tendency to worry.

Diet: Vatas are apt to eat quickly, or very little. They also frequently suffer from digestive difficulties and may have problems with nutrient absorption. Vatas tend to gravitate toward astringent foods, such as salads, but their bodies actually need sweet, sour and salty tastes.

When balanced: vata energy produces feelings of freshness, lightness, happiness and joy. Out of balance, vata produces fear, nervousness, anxiety, tremors and spasms.

To balance vata energy: keep warm and calm; avoid raw foods and cold foods, as well as extremely cold temperatures; eat warm foods cooked with spices and keep a regular routine.

Pitta

Influence: Pitta is the principle of fire.

Physical: Pitta people tend to be of medium height and build, and seldom gain or lose much weight. In general, they are much stronger than vatas. Pittas tend to have bright eyes, which may be gray, green or brown, and a ruddy complexion with silky reddish, blond or light-brown hair. Moles and freckles are common among pittas, who also may have oily, warm skin, and perspire more than others.

Emotional: Pittas tend to have sharp, enterprising minds, but when under stress they demonstrate anger and irritability.

Diet: Pittas crave hot, spicy foods, but these are not good for them. Instead, they should eat foods with sweet, bitter, astringent tastes

When balanced: pitta promotes intelligence and understanding and is crucial to higher learning. Out-of-balance pitta energy may arouse fiery emotions such as anger, hatred, frustration, criticism and jealousy.

To balance pitta: avoid excessive heat, oil and steam; eat nonspicy foods and cool drinks; exercise during the cooler parts of the day.

Kapha

Influence: Kapha combines the energies of water and earth.

Physical: Kaphas tend to have strong, healthy, well-developed bodies. Because their frames may be large, they may carry excess weight. Kaphas have a strong, vital capacity and stamina, and tend to be quite healthy. They may have soft, smooth, oily skin, large dark eyes, strong white teeth and thick, dark, soft, wavy hair. Kaphas tend to be heavy sleepers.

Emotional: Kaphas are slow to anger, and they have a tendency to be possessive and complacent.

Diet: Kaphas have slow digestion and metabolism with a steady appetite and thirst. Kaphas often have a sweet tooth. They also are attracted to salty and oily foods, which they should avoid. Instead, kaphas need bitter, astringent and pungent tastes.

When balanced: kapha energy expresses itself in feelings of love, calmness and forgiveness. Out of balance, kapha creates attachment, greed, lust and envy.

To balance kapha energy: get plenty of exercise; avoid heavy foods; keep active; vary routine; avoid dairy foods, iced food and drinks, and fatty or oily foods. Eat light, dry foods.

Ayurvedic Therapies

Several spas and wellness centers around the country have begun to incorporate Ayurvedic therapies in treatment regimens. You also can use Ayurveda at home to prevent and treat a number of common ailments. Check with your doctor before beginning any complementary therapy. If you get green light, try some of these Ayurvedic remedies.

Anxiety. Feelings of tension and nervousness often derive from a buildup of vata energy in the nervous system. To balance vata energy:

•Soak your way to serenity. To a tub of warm water add 1/2 cup powdered ginger root and 1/3 cup of baking soda. Soak for 15 minutes.
•Make like a corpse. Lie on your back in the yoga posture known as *savasana*, or corpse pose, with your arms by your side. Enjoy the posture as long as you like.
•Say Ommm....Sit quietly, focusing your attention on the crown of your head. Try to meditate for at least 20 minutes twice a day.

Colds and flu may run you down when kapha and vata energies are imbalanced. Your body builds up an excess of cool, moist kapha qualities, resulting in congestion. At the same time, excess vata energy leads to chills, loss of appetite and poor digestion. To speed healing:

•Sip ginger tea. Combine 1 part ginger, 1 part cinnamon and 2 parts lemongrass. Steep 1 tsp. of this mixture in 1 cup hot water for 10 minutes. Strain and add honey, if you wish. Drink up to three cups a day.

Headaches may result from imbalances of several dosha energies. Vata headaches are said to be caused by fear, anxiety, stress and nervousness. Pitta headaches may result if you become overheated or develop acid indigestion. For tension in the neck and shoulders.Kapha headaches may be caused by energy imbalances that lead to sinus congestion. For tension headaches:

•Massage aching muscles with sesame oil.
•Steam away your pain with a hot shower.

Indigestion. That burning sensation from sternum to stomach may an indication that your pitta energy is out of whack. Try this:

•Eat a clove of fresh garlic that you've chopped and mashed with a pinch of salt and baking soda.
•Drink the freshly squeezed juice of 1/4 of a lime, mixed with 1/2 tsp.of baking soda in a cup of warm water.

Insomnia. Grandma also was in synch with Ayurveda if she advised you to:

•Drink a cup of warm milk to which you've added up to 1/8 tsp. of grated nutmeg.
•Try a tea of chamomile, made by steeping 1 tsp. herb in 1 cup hot water for 15 minutes.

Sore Throat. Banish pain and inflammation by:
•Gargling morning and evening with 1 cup hot water mixed with 1/2 tsp....turmeric and 1/2 tsp. salt.
•Avoiding mucus-producing dairy foods.

There's some evidence that chiropractic often helps those people. Could it help you? Discuss the possibility with your physician.

Chiropractic Controvery

Some people swear by chiropractors. Others think they quack louder than Donald Duck. Either way, more than 20 million Americans visit chiropractors each year, most seeking help for back pain, which afflicts up to 90 percent of adults.

Chiropractic—from the Greek for "done by hand"—was born in 1895 after Daniel Palmer, an Iowa grocer, reputedly restored a man's hearing by manipulating his spine. Palmer came up with the notion that nearly all diseases result from nerves pinched by misaligned vertebrae. You have 24 of these moveable bones protecting your spinal cord, and between each are nerves extending to all parts of your body. The spine, Palmer reasoned, was a pathway to the brain. Thus, he theorized, a spinal malformity could cause all sorts of ills.

Chiropractic involves spinal manipulation to treat a variety of ailments. "A problem with just one vertebra can force the entire spine to compensate, putting stress on the other vertebrae and sparking spasms in connecting muscles," says Jerome McAndrews, D.C. (doctor of chiropractic), a spokesman for the American Chiropractic Association in Arlington, Virginia.

Like conventional doctors, chiropractors log two to four years of premedical training. Then they must complete four years of chiropractic college. Most chiropractors employ a variety of diagnostic tools, including orthopedic, neurological and manual examinations, X rays, and, sometimes, magnetic resonance imaging .

Not all chiropractors follow the same treatment procedures. Some stick to spinal manipulation. Some augment spinal therapy with nutritional counseling and holistic healing approaches, such as homeopathy and herbal therapy. And others prescribe more arcane treatments, including electrical stimulation and hot and cold applications.

Most chiropractors work on backs—and there are plenty to keep them busy. Back pain costs Americans $20 million a year in medical and disability payments. In fact, it's the leading reason for doctor visits—although studies show that nine out of 10 back-pain sufferers will recover within a month without any intervention whatsoever.

But after decades of research, no one knows whether back pain results from injuries to muscles, ligaments, disks, bones, or a combination. All conventional doctors can do is to recommend that patients remain as active as possible and take over-the-counter pain relievers and, occasionally, prescription muscle relaxants.

Just a few years ago, the medical community considered most chiropractors to be little more than charlatans. Today, doctors, HMOs and hospitals increasingly refer back-pain patients to chiropractors.

In the last three decades, 17 chiropractic colleges have been accredited in the United States, and the National Institutes of Health has allocated funds to research chiropractic's claims.

That's impressive when you consider that until 1980 the American Medical Association deemed chiropractic an "unscientific cult" and declared it unethical for doctors to refer patients to chiropractors.

Today chiropractors are licensed in all 50 states. Moreover, chiropractic care for back pain is covered under Medicare, worker's compensation, some state Medicaid plans and a growing number of private insurance companies.

"Our main goal is to build a professional bridge with the conventional medical community," McAndrews says. "And I think we're doing that well. In just a few years chiropractic has come a long, long way."

Does Chiropractic Work?

In 1994, after reviewing more than 4,000 studies, the Agency for Health Care Policy and Research, a branch of the federal Department of Health and Human Services, concluded that chiropractic is a safe and effective nondrug treatment for acute lower back pain.

"By manipulating your spine, chiropractors relax back muscles, extend the spine's range of motion and help eliminate pain associated with poor posture," says Scott Haldeman, a conventional physician and chiropractor at the University of California, Irvine College of Medicine.

In addition, more than six published studies suggest that chiropractic is effective in treating neck pain and stiffness. Recently in Quebec, Canada, a medical panel on whiplash-related disorders concluded that spinal manipulation is at least as effective as physical and drug therapies in treating whiplash pain.

Is chiropractic effective for treating other ailments? Maybe. Clay McDonald, D.C., dean of clinics at Palmer College of Chiropractic in Davenport, Iowa, estimates that 30 percent of his patients find chiropractic useful for relieving headache pain.

A 1995 study in the *Journal of Manipulation and Physiological Therapeutics* compared headache patients who underwent six weeks of chiropractic treatment with those who took an antidepressant commonly prescribed for severe headache pain. The researchers concluded that chiropractic patients experienced a 30 percent greater reduction in headache pain and frequency.

But another clinical trial, published in the *Journal of the American Medical Association*, found no evidence that chiropractic was effective at treating tension headaches.

Other advocates of chiropractic swear it works to treat a host of other ills, including asthma, ear infections and even painful menstrual periods.

"But there is no evidence to suggest that chiropractic can cure diabetes, cancer, Parkinson's disease or any other serious disease," Haldeman says. "In fact, seeing a chiropractor can make things worse for individuals suffering from these conditions. How? By discouraging them from getting medical treatments that are of proven effectiveness."

If You See a Chiropractor

Always consult a medical doctor first to determine whether chiropractic can help your condition. Then:

• Look for a chiropractor who treats only musculoskeletal conditions and consults frequently with medical doctors and physical therapists.

• Avoid chiropractors who use jargon like "nerve interference."

• Agree to an initial back X ray. But question the benefit of repeated X rays or full-spine X rays, which doctors say offer little diagnostic benefit.

• Find another practitioner if your chiropractor insists you take nutritional supplements or herbal remedies. Check with your physician before taking anything.

• Ask up front how many sessions you may need. Don't agree to "open-ended" therapy.

Your Eyelids Are Growing Heavy

Since 1958, when the American Medical Association endorsed it as a valid therapy, more health professionals have been recommending hypnosis for a variety of ailments, including lower back pain; migraine headaches; irritable bowel syndrome; burns; multiple sclerosis; fibromyalgia; and pain caused by cancer, arthritis and accidents.

Hypnosis also has been used to relieve symptoms of insomnia, asthma and allergies; stabilize bleeding and blood-sugar levels; lower blood pressure; eradicate warts, blisters and bruises; act as anesthesia during surgery or dental work, and even spur the immune system to accelerate healing.

So why aren't more of us using hypnosis? "The biggest problem with hypnosis is the cultural baggage it carries," says Melvin Gravitz, Ph.D., director of the American Psychological Association's division on hypnotherapy in Washington, D.C.

Modern medical hypnotists, Gravitz says, bear little resemblance to the Svengali-like characters popularized by Hollywood films, or Las Vegas lounge performers who prompt audience members to cluck like

Many people have been able to lose weight, stop smoking and eradicate pain after visiting a hypnotist. Consider seeing one yourself.

chickens. "When used responsibly," Gravitz says, "hypnosis is a very powerful tool."

And most of us—75 percent—can be hypnotized to reap therapeutic benefits, say experts at the American Society of Clinical Hypnosis in Des Plaines, Illinois.

"The greater a person's capacity for imagination, and the more willing she is to enter hypnosis, the greater the chances of success," says Fred Frankel, MD, professor emeritus of psychiatry at Harvard Medical School.

When you undergo hypnosis you simply shift to a state of mind that's relaxed, focused and receptive to suggestions. And it's important to remember that those suggestions must be compatible with your goals and desires. In other words, you'll never quack while in a trance—unless you want to.

"Hypnosis is not unlike daydreaming or being so caught up in a good book that the rest of the world falls away," says Stephen Lankton, a Pensacola, Florida, hypnotherapist and president of the American Hypnosis Board for Clinical Social Workers.

But hypnosis is more than just a relaxation tool, says Herbert Benson, M.D., a pioneer in mind-body research at Harvard Medical School. The process triggers profound physiological changes, prompting your body to lower blood pressure, heart and respiratory rates-and to quell pain that may have plagued you for years.

How? Hypnotic trances not only divert your mind from pain, but also blunt pain signals and prevent them from setting off alarms in your brain, says John Baren, a clinical social worker who hypnotizes pain patients in Centerville, Ohio. In addition, Baren says, hypnosis may increase levels of endorphins and enkaphalins, the body's natural painkillers.

In the last few decades, hundreds of studies have pointed out the benefits of using hypnosis to control pain. One of the most conclusive took place at Virginia Polytechnic Institute and State University in Blacksburg.

Helen Crawford, Ph.D, a professor of experimental psychology, found that 70 percent of patients who practiced self-hypnosis for three weeks were able to reduce back pain significantly. Whenever patients felt discomfort, they were asked to imagine themselves in a peaceful place or to envision flipping a switch to shut off pain.

Another study, at Albert Einstein College of Medicine in New York, suggests that hypnosis may have profound effects on the body's immune system. Researchers Marcia Greenleaf and Stanley Fisher noted that coronary bypass patients who accepted hypnotic suggestions recovered far more quickly than patients who received no trance therapy.

Could you benefit from hypnosis? Probably, says Dr. John A. Scott, Jr., a psychologist in Memphis, Tennessee . "Hypnosis is a way of tuning into what's going on inside you and responding to your deepest issues," he says. "When you do that you can become very focused and responsive-maybe in ways that would amaze you."

Hypnotize Yourself

It's easy practice hypnosis at home, says D. Corydon Hammond, PhD, a therapist in Salt Lake City, Utah, and past president of the American Society of Clinical Hypnotists. Here's how:

•Sit in a comfortable chair and close your eyes. Focus on your breathing. Take slow, deep breaths without pausing.
•As you inhale, think, 'calm.' With each exhalation, think 'relax.'
•After three minutes, mentally give yourself a positive suggestion, using imagery. See yourself, for example, as being pain free and full of joy.
•Slowly repeat the suggestion three times, or allow your mind to retain the positive image for up to 30 seconds.
•Finish by counting backward from 10 to 0, as you gradually become aware of your surroundings.

Or try this method endorsed by therapists at Albert Einstein College of Medicine in New York City:

•Look up, as if trying to see the top of your head.
•As you continue to look up, close your eyes slowly. Take a deep breath and hold it to a count of three.
•Exhale and let your eyes relax, as you imagine your body floating.
•Give yourself a positive suggestion, using imagery.

To come out of your trance:
•With your eyes still closed, look up.
•Open your eyes slowly, allowing them to focus.

Perhaps you're among the 25 percent or so of people who fail to enter a hypnotic state. Perhaps the thought of sipping a tea made from Chinese lizards leaves you feeling a little queasy. There are scores of complementary medicines out there and sooner or later you'll find one that suits your needs. Or maybe not.

Find What Works for You

The point is that it's up to you to maintain your health, in whatever way works best for you. It's your body. It's your mind. It's certainly your spirit. Take responsibility for yourself.

Sure, we all backslide from time to time. Life would be exceedingly boring if we didn't. Enjoy those greasy fries once in a while, but don't forsake the vegetables and fruits. Kick back on the couch and catch a flick, but remember to take a walk later. Lose your cool in traffic if you must, but spend the next five minutes breathing deeply.

Achieving health and maintaining your new lifestyle are goals within the reach of almost anyone. It's simple, it's easy and you can do it.

Remember, health is a journey. Have a good one. Live healthy, now and forever!

Staying Healthy Action Plan

•**Explore your options**. If you develop a health problem, don't just take a prescription drug without considering an alternative. Discuss complementary therapies with your doctor.

•**Pinpoint your problem.** If you suffer from pain, nausea, asthma or other chronic problems, consider acupuncture. The federal government considers it a safe, effective treatment for many ailments.

•**Apply some pressure**. If needles turn you off, you can still benefit from the principles of acupuncture. Check out a book on acupressure and try massaging away your health-related worries.

•**Trance out**. See a hypnotist. Hypnosis is effective for relieving insomnia, addictions, hypertension and other health problems. It is worth a try.

•**Surf the web.** Visit a chat room and ask others how they've dealt with an ailment. Look for web sites dealing with complementary therapies. Have an open mind.

Appendix

Natural Therapies at a Glance

To achieve and maintain good health it's important to see your doctor regularly. But remember that ultimately it is your responsibility to take care of yourself. Eat well, exercise, meditate, get plenty of sleep and don't forget to have fun. In addition, don't overlook the many ways that you can care for yourself at home.

Always check first with your doctor before trying a home remedy. If your doctor agrees, consider these simple solutions to common health problems.

Anxiety

In our stress-filled world, anxiety is something we all experience from time to time. Symptoms may include nervousness, inability to concentrate, muscle tension, heart palpitations, dry mouth, excessive sweating, irritability and insomnia. Untreated, anxiety may contribute to a number of physical ailments, including heart disease.

Prevention

Keep yourself in good physical health and you likely will be emotionally healthy as well.

Eat a balanced diet rich in nutrients.

Get plenty of exercise and sleep.

If your schedule is too hectic, take steps to lighten the load.

Treatment

Acupressure: To calm your nerves and reduce feelings of uneasiness, place your thumb in the center of your inner wrist, two fingers width from the wrist crease and between the two bones of your forearm. Press firmly for one minute. Do this three to five times, then repeat on the other arm.

Aromatherapy: Essential oils of lavender (*Lavandula officinalis*), jasmine (*Jasminum officinale*) and chamomile (*Matricaria recutita*) may help you to relax. Put a drop or two on a tissue and inhale. Rub the oils into your temples. Or add 5 to 6 drops to a steam inhalation or bath.

Exercise: Exercise promotes blood circulation, and produces endorphins, the body's natural tranquilizers and pain killers.

Herbs: Take teas, tinctures or capsules of mildly calming herbs, including chamomile, lemon balm (*Melissa officinalis*) and linden (*tilia spp*). Stronger herbs such as skullcap (*Scutellaria lateriflora*), valerian (*Valeriana officinalis*), hops (*Humulus lupulus*) and passionflower (*Passiflora incarnata*) may help to relieve anxiety-induced insomnia.

Meditation: If your muscles are tense or aching, try progressive muscle relaxation, easing tension in your muscles, one by one. Sit quietly and breathe deeply for 15 minutes at least twice a day.

Nutrition: Eat a well-balanced diet rich in nutrients. Avoid drugs such as alcohol, and reduce or eliminate consumption of sugar and caffeine.

Supplements: Magnesium supplements also may help you to deal with anxiety.

Yoga: Lie on your back in a comfortable place. Inhale slowly through your nose, using your diaphragm (allowing your abdomen to expand). Take in as much air as possible. Breathe out, reversing the diaphragm pressure (allowing your stomach to contract). Repeat the exercise several times.

Arthritis

Arthritis encompasses a wide variety of disorders, but generally refers to degenerative joint disease. Arthritis may result from disease, injury, infection, genetic defect or some other cause.

Prevention
Exercise regularly.
Avoid injuries that may stress your joints.
Eat collagen-producing foods.

Treatment
Acupressure: Manipulating various pressure points may help you, depending on your symptoms. Press the point on your spine between the

third and fourth thoracic vertebrae, approximately at shoulder level. Also try pressing the point on the outside border of your calf, in the depression between the tibia and fibula bones. Or press the point three inches below the dimple or depression on the outside of your knee, approximately an inch from the crest of the shinbone, in a groove or natural depression in a muscle.

Aromatherapy: Apply to affected areas oils of chamomile, camphor (*Cinnamomum camphora*), eucalyptus (*Eucalyptus globulus*), lavender or rosemary (*Rosemarinus officinalis*).

Exercise: Try swimming or other water exercises in a heated pool. Water supports the body and can reduce stress so that you can work on moving affected joints.

Herbs: To relieve pain, try white willow bark (*Salix albica*), black cohosh (*Cimifuga racemosa*) or nettle (*Urtica dioica*). To relieve muscle tension, rub affected areas with tinctures of lobelia (*Lobelia inflata*) and cramp bark (*Viburnum opulus*). Ointments containing cayenne (*Capsicum frutescens*) increase blood circulation and ease pain of affected areas.

Meditation: Meditation, self-hypnosis, guided imagery, and relaxation techniques can help to control pain.

Nutrition: To lessen arthritic symptoms tied to allergies, avoid foods such as grains, nuts, meats, eggs and dairy products. Also eliminate vegetables in the nightshade family (tomato, potato, eggplant and pepper). The alkaloids in these foods may inhibit formation of collagen, which you need to make joint cartilage. Eat cherries or dark red berries to stimulate collagen production To ease the pain and inflammation of rheumatoid arthritis, stick to a low-fat, low-protein vegetarian diet. Researchers in Norway found that rheumatoid arthritics who eliminated meat, eggs, dairy products, sugar and foods with gluten, such as wheat bread, improved dramatically within a month. Also eliminate partially hydrogenated fats and polyunsaturated vegetable oils. Supplement your diet instead with flax oil, sardines and other oily fish, which are a source of omega-3 fatty acids.

Supplements: Many arthritics have found relief by taking supplements such as glucosamine and chondroitin sulfate.

Yoga: To loosen joints in your hand, do the Spider Push-Up. Press your fingertips together firmly, palms two to three inches apart. Push palms toward each other while touching your fingertips. Do this 20 times. To ease stiff finger joints, do the Thumb Squeeze. Curl your fingers into a fist around your thumb. Gently squeeze and slowly release. Do this 10 times with each hand. Stretch hips and back with the Dog and Cat. On your hands and knees (like a table), inhale as you lower your back and lift your head and buttocks (Dog). Then exhale as you arch your back and drop your head and buttocks (Cat). Do this nine times.

Cholesterol Problems

Nearly half of all Americans—40 percent—have cholesterol levels that physicians consider to be unhealthy. Cholesterol can clog your arteries, putting you at risk for heart attacks and strokes.

Prevention
Maintain a healthy body weight.
Eat a nutritionally balanced diet, with no more than 300 mg a day of cholesterol.
Quit smoking.
Have your cholesterol level checked regularly. Home test kits are available.

Treatment
Aromatherapy: Inhaling essential oil of rosemary may help to normalize high blood cholesterol, according to some aromatherapists.
Exercise: Exercise by itself may not lower total cholesterol, but exercising moderately several times a week raises levels of beneficial cholesterol.
Herbs: Try garlic (*Allium sativa*), turmeric (*Curcuma longa*), ginseng (*Panax ginseng*) and fenugreek (*Trigonell foenum-graecum*).
Meditation: Stress may contribute to elevated cholesterol levels. Try relaxation techniques such as meditation, visualization and guided imagery.
Nutrition: Avoid saturated fats derived from animal products and tropical oils. Fat should comprise no more than 30 percent of your daily diet. Eat more fruits, vegetables and whole grains, which are cholesterol free and rich in artery-cleansing fiber. A compound found in grape skin products, including wine, lowers cholesterol.
Supplements: Try vitamin E. Research also indicates that vitamin C raises level of beneficial cholesterol.

Colds and Flu

Both colds and influenza are caused by viruses. There are more than 200 such viruses and antibiotics are useless in treating your symptoms.

Prevention
Keep your immune system in tip-top shape by eating a nutritionally balanced diet, and drinking plenty of water every day, at least eight eight-ounce glasses.
Stay away from people who have been infected with cold or flu viruses.
Wash your hands frequently.

Treatment

Acupressure: To support your respiratory system, press your thumb into your solar plexus/diaphragm and massage for a few seconds.

Aromatherapy: Add a few drops of the oils of eucalyptus, wintergreen (*Gaultheria procumbens*) or peppermint (*Mentha piperita*) to a bowl of boiling water. Place a towel over your head and breathe.

Exercise: Walking 45 minutes a day may boost your immune system and help you to recover faster.

Herbs: Taken at the first sign of symptoms, echinacea (*Echinacea spp*) and garlic may reduce the intensity and duration of your illness by stimulating your immune system. Ginger (*Zingiber officinalis*) will warm you up and banish nausea.

Nutrition: Clinical evidence supports the folk notion that chicken soup is healing; chemical constituents of the soup keep neutrophils from clumping and causing inflammation. Eating chili or other spicy foods containing horseradish, hot pepper sauce, hot mustard or curry will help to break up congestion. Avoid dairy products, which thicken mucus.

Supplements: Try vitamins A and C, along with B-complex vitamins, as well minerals zinc and copper.

Constipation

Constipation may be caused by not eating enough fiber, not drinking enough water, not getting enough exercise, or by emotional or psychological problems caused by stress.

Prevention

Don't drink too much coffee, tea or alcohol; all are dehydrating and can lead to constipation.

Avoid milk and cheese if you're constipated. Both contain casein, an insoluble protein that may bind your intestinal tract.

Treatment

Acupressure: Press the point that corresponds with your large intestine. You'll find it in the web between your thumb and index finger. Do this one minute and repeat. Do not do this exercise if you are pregnant.

Aromatherapy: Inhaling and/or massaging your abdomen with any of these essential oils may help to relieve your symptoms: black pepper (*Piper nigrum*), camphor, fennel (*Foeniculum vulgare*), marjoram (*Origanum marjorana*) or rose (*Rose spp*).

Nutrition: Add more fiber to your diet. Fiber cleanses your colon. The American Dietetic Association recommends that most people consume 30 grams of fiber a day. Fresh rhubarb also may relieve constipation.

Supplements: Try supplements containing psyllium.

Yoga: The Cobra position is one of the best positions for nurturing your abdominal organs. Lie on your stomach with your legs together and the side of your head resting on the floor. Keep your palms beneath your shoulders, your elbows close to your body. Inhale and lift your head and chest off the floor, face forward. Your navel should touch the floor. Look as high as you can. Hold the position for three to six seconds. Then exhale and slowly come back down. Do this four times a day.

Coughs

A cough is a protective reflex that kicks in when the membranes lining your respiratory tract secrete excessive mucus or phlegm. The most common cause of coughs is an acute respiratory tract infection.

Prevention
Eat a healthy, nutrition-rich diet.
Drink plenty of water every day.
Exercise regularly.
Avoid people who have colds or flu.

Treatment
Acupressure: Bend your left elbow and make a fist. Place your right thumb on the outside crease of the elbow, along the taut tendon. Press for one minute. Repeat on the other arm. Do this three times.

Aromatherapy: Rub your throat with the essential oils of eucalyptus or myrrh (*Commiphora molmol*).

Herbs: Try coltsfoot (*Tussilago farfara*), marsh mallow (*Althea officinalis*), hyssop (*Hyssopus officinalis*) anise (*Pimpinella anisum*) or licorice (*Glycyrrhiza glabra*).

Nutrition: Drink fresh fruit and vegetable juices. Eat a well-balanced diet.

Supplements: Take vitamin C.

Depression

Depression is a mood disorder lasting at least two weeks, which produces exaggerated feelings of sadness, worthlessness, emptiness and dejection.

Prevention
Eat a nutritious, well-balanced diet.
Exercise regularly.
Don't overwork yourself.

Develop hobbies.
Take regular vacations.

Treatment
Acupressure: Bend your right knee and place your thumb above the inside knee crease, just below the joint. Press for one minute. Do this three times on each leg.

Aromatherapy: Essential oils of basil (*Occimum basilicum*), clary (*Salvia sclarea*), jasmine, rose and chamomile may ease mental fatigue.

Exercise: Exercise improves blood flow to the brain, elevates mood and relieves stress. Studies show that jogging for 30 minutes three times a week can be as effective as psychotherapy at treating mild depression.

Herbs: There have been at least 16 randomized, double-blind studies comparing St. John's wort (*Hypericum perforatum*) with a placebo. In 13 of those studies, researchers noted a statistically significant improvement among patients who took the herb.

Meditation: Meditation, progressive relaxation techniques, visualization and guided imagery may help to reduce stress and elevate your mood.

Nutrition: Avoid alcohol, junk food, sugar, aspartame, and caffeine. Eat foods containing the calming amino acid tryptophan, including turkey, chicken, fish, cooked dried beans and peas, brewers yeast, peanut butter, nuts and soybeans. Eat carbohydrates to encourage brain uptake of tryptophan.

Supplements: Some studies indicate that depression may be relieved by taking the vitamin B complex, folic acid, S-adenosylmethionene (SAMe) and the antioxidant selenium.

Diarrhea

Diarrhea may be caused by consuming too much rich food, coffee, or fruit, or it may result from stress or other illnesses, including flu, irritable bowel syndrome, diverticulitis, colitis, Crohn's disease, AIDS and cancer.

Prevention
Stay away from foods that disagree with you.
Reduce stress, which may contribute to diarrhea.

Treatment
Aromatherapy: Inhaling and/or massaging your abdomen with any of these essential oils may help to relieve your symptoms: black pepper, chamomile, camphor, cypress, eucalyptus, geranium, lavender, myrrh,, neroli (*Citrus aurantium*), peppermint, rosemary or sandalwood (*Santalum album*).

Herbs: Drink teas of peppermint or chamomile to ease intestinal spasms and cramps.

Nutrition: Eat a well-balanced diet and drink plenty of water to make up for fluids lost from diarrhea. Drink only clear liquids, such as soda, tea, bouillon and apple juice. Glucose has a binding effect on your system. Add a teaspoon of sugar to tea or apple juice. Eat live yogurt, whose cultures contain bacteria your bowels will have lost after a bout with diarrhea.

Enlarged Prostate

Most men over the age of 60 have some symptoms associated with benign prostatic hyperplasia, or BPH. Left untreated, BPH can lead to dangerous complications, including bladder and kidney infections, and prostate cancer.

Prevention
Take warm sitz baths.
Drink more water; dehydration stresses the prostate.
Avoid prolonged bicycle riding, horseback riding, or other exercises that may irritate the prostate.
Take supplements of zinc and vitamin C.

Treatment
Herbs: Several studies show that saw palmetto berries work faster and better than Proscar, a leading pharmaceutical drug.

Massage: Massage the prostate or have sex more often. Ejaculation empties the prostate of secretions that may hamper urination.

Nutrition: Avoid alcohol, which tightens the bladder neck and encourages urination. Avoid spicy and acidic foods if they give you problems.

Supplements: Zinc is involved with many aspects of hormonal metabolism, and may promote prostate health and reduce inflammation. Also beneficial to the prostate are vitamins C and E, the amino acids glycine, alanine and glutamic acid.

Yoga: Try the Boat Posture. Inhale as you lift your head, chest, arms and legs off the floor. Stretch your arms behind you and hold the position for 15 seconds. Then exhale as you relax back onto the floor. Do either or both exercises twice a day.

High Blood Pressure

High blood pressure, also known as hypertension, is the most common form of all cardiovascular disease in the western world and the leading cause of strokes.

Prevention
Eat a healthy, balanced diet.
Exercise regularly.
Lose weight, if you need to do so.
Don't start smoking.
Don't drink alcohol excessively.

Treatment

Acupressure: Using your thumb, apply firm pressure for one minute at the point along your biceps tendon at the elbow crease, in a direct line with your ring finger. Repeat on the other arm.

Aromatherapy: Inhale or add to your bath any of these soothing essential oils: clary, hyssop, lavender, lemon balm, marjoram (*Origanum marjorana*) or ylang-ylang (*Canaga odorata*).

Exercise: The best type of exercise for people with high blood pressure is an aerobic activity, such as walking, jogging, cycling or swimming. Avoid weight lifting or other isometric exercises that cause you to strain.

Herbs: One of the best herbs you can take for high blood pressure is hawthorn (*Cratageus laevigata*). Several studies have shown that hawthorn normalizes blood pressure. A great deal of clinical research supports the use of garlic by hypertensives.

Massage: Massage may help to lower your blood pressure by "teaching" your body how to relax. Particularly helpful is shiatsu, a form of Japanese massage that focuses on pressure points used by acupuncturists and acupressurists.

Meditation: Practicing mediation on a regular basis can help you to relax and lower your blood pressure. Try guided imagery and visualization—imagining your blood pressure falling—and see if it really does go down.

Nutrition: Eat a diet that is high in fiber and low in salt and fat. Form your diet around fruits, vegetables and whole grains. Fatty acids found in fish also are good for you because they relax arteries and thin the blood. Avoid salt, which contains sodium and cause you to retain fluid, which raises pressure. Consume caffeine and alcohol moderately, if at all.

Supplements: Potassium is especially important for lowering blood pressure. Several studies suggest that calcium and/or magnesium may help some people with high blood pressure.

Yoga: Yoga is a great form of exercise for people with high blood pressure. Most poses are deeply relaxing. But avoid poses such as head stands that cause blood to rush to your head.

Indigestion

Excess stomach acid may be caused by stress, overeating (especially rich or spicy foods that don't agree with you), overindulging in alcohol, obesity, smoking or using analgesics such as aspirin.

Prevention

Maintain a healthy weight.
Don't overeat, especially foods rich in fat.
Avoid spicy foods.
Don't drink too much alcohol.
Stop smoking.
Reduce stress in your life.

Treatment

Aromatherapy: Inhale, add to a bath or massage your abdomen and sternum with any of these essential oils: basil, chamomile, fennel, lavender, peppermint.

Herbs: Try meadowsweet (*Filipendula ulmaria*), lavender, chamomile or peppermint.

Nutrition: Avoid junk foods and foods that don't agree with you. Substitute herbal teas for coffee. Each a well-balanced, nutritious diet rich in vegetables and fruits. Eat balanced portions. Chew your food slowly and thoroughly before swallowing.

Headaches

Tension headaches may be caused by stress, as well as anxiety, persistent noise, eyestrain, poor posture or excessive consumption of caffeine. Vascular headaches, which include migraine and cluster headaches, are caused by constricted blood vessels. Migraines may be triggered by excessive caffeine, various foods or scents, dry winds, changes in altitude and seasons, hormonal fluctuations, or missing a meal. Cluster headaches are more common among heavy smokers and drinkers.

In addition, headaches may be caused or aggravated by colds, flu, sinus problems, hay fever and other seasonal allergies.

Prevention

Avoid foods that don't agree with you.
Reduce stress in your life.
Avoid noisy, smoky places.

Treatment

General headache relief: Place your index fingers at the top of each foot, fingertips next to the large knuckle of the big toe, between the big and second toes. Press for one minute and release. Repeat two to three times twice daily. Or, place the tip of your middle finger at the top of the bridge of your nose, between your eyebrows. Press lightly for two minutes and breathe deeply. Repeat three to five times at least twice a day.

Aromatherapy: Try oils of lavender, eucalyptus, wintergreen (*Gaultheria procumbens*), rosemary or peppermint.

Exercise: Regular exercise releases endorphins, the body's natural pain killers, and helps to dilate blood vessels, which may prevent migraines.

Herbs: Feverfew (*Chrysanthemum parthenium*) dilates constricted blood vessels, which can cause headaches, especially migraines. Also helpful are hawthorn, linden and skullcap (*Scutellaria lateriflora*).

Massage: Give yourself a scalp massage. Place both middle fingers on your forehead at the hairline. Using gentle pressure, gradually work your fingers back to the crown of your head. Repeat in half-inch increments until you reach your temples. Rotate your fingers on both sides for a few minutes. Then bring your thumbs to the base of your skull along your hairline, and massage both sides of your skull up to the crown.

Meditation: Meditation and guided relaxation therapies are helpful in reducing stress that may cause tension headaches. While seated, breathe deeply and think calming thoughts. Inhale and gently tip your head back until you are looking at the ceiling. Exhale and bring your head forward until your chin rests on your chest. Repeat twice.

Nutrition: Avoid foods that can cause migraines, including chocolate, aged cheeses, citrus fruits, processed meats containing sodium nitrates, citrus fruits, red wine, and the food additive MSG.

Supplements: Some people have benefited from taking magnesium and niacin (vitamin B3).

Infections

Your immune system is your body's defense department. When the immune system is alerted to the presence of pathogenic invaders, it calls out a veritable army of infection fighters. Proteins called antibodies team up with special white blood cells to neutralize and destroy pathogens. When white blood cells called neutrophils clump together at infection sites, you experience the achiness and inflammation that accompany infections.

Prevention
Don't eat foods you suspect may have been infected by germs.
Wash your hands regularly.
Avoid dirt and filth.

Treatment

Aromatherapy: Inhale and/or add to a bath antiseptic oil of lavender.

Herbs: Echinacea holds promise as a treatment for some viral conditions, such as colds and flu, because it significantly boosts your body's immune system and helps you to heal faster than you otherwise might. Another major antiseptic and antibiotic herb is garlic.

Meditation: Some studies indicate that infections may be reduced or eliminated by visualizing your white cells attacking invading pathogens. Be sure to get plenty of rest when battling an infection.

Nutrition: Keep your immune system in good shape by eating foods high in nutritional value, including whole grains, vegetables and fruits and low-fat dairy products.

Insomnia

Inability to fall asleep or stay asleep is one of the most common complaints in our culture today.

Prevention
Eat a healthy diet.
Get plenty of exercise, but not directly before bedtime.
Meditate.

Treatment

Exercise: Calming exercises, including yoga, also promote sleep.

Herbs: Try valerian, chamomile or skullcap.

Meditation: Sit calmly in a quiet room, your hands on your knees. Breathe deeply and regularly and try to clear your mind of thoughts. Do this for 20 minutes.

Nutrition: Because high or low blood sugar levels may disrupt sleep patterns, avoid sweets and fruit juices before bed. To activate sedative neurotransmitters in your brain, each starchy food—a plain baked potato or a slice of bread—half an hour before bed. Also try drinking warm milk, which contains the calming amino acid tryptophan.

Supplements: Try melatonin, calcium or magnesium.

Menopause

Menopause is not a disease; it's a natural part of a woman's life and there's no way to prevent it. In menopause the body produces less estrogen, which increases risk of osteoporosis. Menopause also may bring about a rise in blood cholesterol levels, leaving you at risk for developing heart attacks or strokes.

Treatment

Aromatherapy: Inhale or add to a bath essential oils of chamomile, cypress or fennel. .

Exercise: Practice weight-bearing exercises to avoid osteoporosis.

Herbs: Several herbs contain chemicals called phytoestrogens. These chemicals perform like natural estrogen, but without the side effects. Try angelica (*Angelica sinensis*), ginseng (*Panax ginseng*) or black cohosh (*Cimicifuga racemosa*).

Nutrition: Eat foods high in plant estrogens, such as soy beans, lima beans, nuts and seeds, fennel, celery, parsley and flaxseed oil.

Supplements: Take calcium to prevent osteoporosis. Vitamin E may help to treat hot flashes and reduce risk of cardiovascular disease.

Muscle Pain

Muscle pain may be caused by overexertion, muscle cramps, strained muscles, whiplash after an accident, influenza, drug reactions, fibromyalgia and polymyalgia. Fortunately, it's easy to treat muscle pain naturally.

Prevention

Don't try to take on more physical activity than you can handle.

Be cautious when lifting or carrying; always "lift with your legs, not your back."

Take frequent breaks during strenuous physical activity.

If possible, avoid drugs such as corticosteroids, which may cause muscle pain by depleting your body of potassium.

Avoid heavy blankets and tight pajamas when sleeping.

Treatment

Aromatherapy: For sprained muscles massage affected area or add to a bath essential oils of camphor, eucalyptus, lavender or rosemary.

Herbs: Ointments containing arnica (*Arnica montana*) help to soothe aching muscles and heal bruises. Also helpful are ointments containing capsaicin, which brings warmth to your skin and is found in cayenne pepper.

Massage: Massage helps to push acids out of your muscles. Reduce muscle cramps by rubbing affected area upward, toward the heart.

Nutrition: Drinking a 12-oz glass of tonic water (which contains quinine) at bedtime may reduce the frequency of muscle cramps. Drink sports beverages that contain electrolyte/carbohydrate replacements.

Supplements: Try calcium, magnesium or vitamin E.

Nausea

Although it's usually caused by a digestive problem or an infection, such an influenza, nausea can result in hormonal and other imbalances during pregnancy, or from motion sickness.

Prevention

Avoid rich, spicy foods, or foods that don't agree with you.
Sit in the front seat if you get carsick.
Don't read while riding.
Wear a sea band if you take a cruise.

Treatment

Acupressure: Apply pressure to the inside of your wrist, near the center. Hold for a minute. Then repeat a few times. Sea bands, the bracelets some people wear on cruises, also massage this point, which acupressurists say controls the urge to vomit.

Aromatherapy: Inhale, add to a bath or massage abdomen with any of these essential oils: basil, fennel, lavender, lemon balm, peppermint, rose or sandalwood.

Herbs: Ginger is a well-documented remedy for nausea, especially if it's caused by motion sickness. Also good for nausea are teas made from chamomile, lemon balm or peppermint.

Meditation: Relaxing in a dark quiet room may help to ease feelings of nausea. Guided meditations have helped cancer patients to overcome nausea associated with chemotherapy.

Nutrition: Eat bland foods that don't upset your stomach. Drink plenty of fluids. Avoid milk products, which are more difficult to digest than other foods.

Premenstrual Syndrome

In the 10 to 14 days leading up to your period, you may develop premenstrual syndrome (PMS), with symptoms such as nervousness, mood swings, bloating, headaches, depression, sugar craving, irritability and weight gain.

Prevention

Lessen symptoms by living a healthy lifestyle.

Treatment

Aromatherapy: To ease anxiety and irritability add to your bath 5 drops of oils of lavender or chamomile. To reduce breast tenderness, add to your bath 8 drops of oil geranium.

Herbs: Angelica balances body hormones and has a tonic effect on the uterus. Dandelion leaves (*Taraxacum officinale*) leaves are diuretic and may relieve bloating. Skullcap calms the nerves.

Exercise: Several studies show that regular exercise alleviates symptoms of PMS by stimulating release of endorphins, the body's natural pain killers.

Massage: Gently massaging your abdomen may help to ease the pain of cramps.

Meditation: Relaxing in a quiet, dark room or following a guided meditation may help to relieve your symptoms.

Nutrition: Reduce your consumption of caffeine, sugar, salt, dairy products and white flour, which can aggravate your symptoms. Eating six or more small meals a day may reduce symptoms by keeping insulin levels more constant. Avoid fatty foods. Replace butter with polyunsaturated oils such as flaxseed, corn and safflower. Avoid salty foods, which can contribute to water retention. Counter food cravings with carbohydrates, such as whole grains, pasta and cereal

Supplements: Mood swings, fluid retention, bloatedness, breast tenderness, food cravings and fatigue have been linked to deficiencies of vitamin B6 or magnesium. Also beneficial are supplements of calcium, zinc, copper and vitamins A and E.

Yoga: Try the Bow to restore hormonal balance. Lie on your stomach, legs bent, and grasp both ankles. As you inhale, squeeze your buttocks and slowly raise your head, chest and thighs off the floor. Hold for 15 seconds, breathing slowly, and release.

Sore Throat

At least 90 percent of sore throats are caused by inflammation of throat tissue, often triggered by viral infections, including colds, flu, measles, chickenpox, herpes and mononucleosis.

Prevention

Replace your toothbrush once a month; bacteria tend to collect on the bristles.

Avoid people who have colds or flu.

Stay healthy by eating a balanced, nutritious diet.

Take a multivitamin every day.

Treatment

Acupressure: Using your left thumb, apply pressure to the center of the pad at the base of your right thumb. Hold for one minute and repeat on the other hand.

Aromatherapy: Inhale or massage throat with any of these essential oils: clary, eucalyptus, geranium or lavender.

Herbs : Garlic is a natural antibiotic and antiseptic. Also try goldenseal (*Hydrastis canadensis*), echinacea, sage (*Salvia officinalis*) or slippery elm (*Ulmus fulva*).

Supplements: Try vitamin C and zinc.

Sunburn

If you expose yourself for too long to the sun's ultraviolet rays, your skin could burn, turning red and developing painful blisters. Repeated overexposure can cause your skin to become leathery and dark. And it increases your risk of eventually developing skin cancer.

Prevention

Limit your exposure to direct sunlight, especially during peak hours of 10 a.m. to 3 p.m.

Wear sunscreen.

Be cautious around water, whose surface reflects the sun's rays.

Wear sunglasses.

Treatment

Aromatherapy: Soothing oils such as chamomile and peppermint.

Herbs: Lotions, poultices and compresses containing calendula (*Calendula officinalis*) will reduce inflammation. Preparations containing aloe (*Aloe barbadensis*) are excellent for dryness and irritation.

Nutrition: Eat foods high in vitamin E, including whole grains and vegetable oils

Supplements: Taking vitamin E supplements may decrease the inflammation caused by sunburn.

Toothache

Toothaches may be caused by dental disorders, including tooth decay and gum disease. Tooth decay is caused by dental plaque, a substance composed of bacteria, acids and sugars in your mouth, which corrodes the protective enamel of your teeth.

Prevention

Brush and floss your teeth regularly.

Use a cavity-preventing toothpaste with fluoride.

Cut down on sweets and carbohydrates.

Get your teeth cleaned professionally every six months.

Treatment
Acupressure: Apply deep pressure to the webbing between the index finger and thumb. Massaging this area with an ice cube also may help to relieve pain. Don't do this if you're pregnant.

Aromatherapy: Inhale any of these essential oils: chamomile, camphor or peppermint.

Herbs: To numb a painful tooth rub it with oil of clove (*Syzgium aromaticum*) or myrrh (*Commiphora molmol*).

Meditation: Listening to soothing music and practicing deep-breathing exercises may help to alleviate some toothache pains.

Wounds

Cuts usually have clean edges, may bleed a lot and damage muscles, tendons and nerves.

Lacerations have jagged edges and are likely to be more damaging to deep tissue than a cut. Your risk of incurring infections or scarring is greater with lacerations. Scrapes and abrasions occur when you skin is rubbed against a hard surface, breaking small blood vessels in the skin. These are easily contaminated by bacteria. A puncture is a narrow, deep hole produced by a penetrating object. Punctures rarely bleed heavily but may become infected by tetanus and other infections.

Prevention
Avoid dump sites and other areas with broken glass or sharp metal.

To prevent infections, wash all cuts thoroughly with soap and water and apply disinfectant.

Treatment
Aromatherapy: Tea tree oil (*Melaleuca spp*) is antiseptic. Also helpful are any of these essential oils: benzoin (*Styrax benzoin*), bergamot (*Citrus bergamia*), eucalyptus, frankincense, hyssop, juniper (*Juniperus communis*), and patchouli (*Pogostemon patchouli*).

Herbs: Aloe is soothing to skin and may help to prevent scars from forming. Also helpful are ointments containing calendula.

Nutrition: Pineapple contains a substance called bromelain that may reduce inflammation.

Supplements: To speed healing, take vitamin E supplements and/or apply vitamin E oil to the wound. Also helpful are vitamins A, C, and the B complex, as well as the amino acids arginine and glycine taken between meals.

Index

INDEX